MASTERING RISK ASSESSMENT IN HEALTH AND SOCIAL CARE

Protecting Lives and Improving Care

BY

DANIEL MEGUILLE

E-Book: 979-8-9970285-6-5
Paperback: 979-8-9970285-7-2
Hardcover: 979-8-9970285-8-9

Table of Contents

Preface

Navigating the intricate and often challenging landscape of health and social care demands more than just technical knowledge or procedural adherence; it requires a fundamental understanding of the delicate balance between safety and dignity, protection and autonomy. This book, ***"Mastering Risk Assessment in Health and Social Care: Protecting Life, improving Care"***, emerges from a deep-seated commitment to empower practitioners across the sector to face this duality with confidence, wisdom, and compassion. Whether you are a frontline care provider, a manager overseeing complex systems, or a regulatory agent entrusted with safeguarding standards, this work aims to be your steadfast companion in mastering the art and science of risk assessment.

Risk, by its very nature, is a complex and multifaceted concept. It silently permeates every corner of health and social care environments, threading through daily routines, decisions, and interactions. These are spaces where vulnerability intersects with resilience and where choices impact not only safety but the very essence of a person's independence and identity. In this context, risk assessment is far more than a box-ticking exercise or a bureaucratic mandate; it is a dynamic process central to delivering care that is safe yet respectful, protective yet enabling. The tension between guarding against harm and promoting agency calls for a nuanced approach, one that recognises risk as both a hazard to be managed and an opportunity for growth and empowerment.

This book sets out to unravel the complexities of risk assessment through a carefully structured journey, beginning with foundational concepts and advancing toward practical application and cultural transformation. At its heart lies the recognition that effective risk management is rooted in knowledge, legal understanding, and ethical reflection, but it also flourishes through continuous learning, communication, and collaboration. It is about building a culture where risk is openly acknowledged and thoughtfully addressed, not feared or avoided, and where all voices, especially those of the service users at the core of care, are valued and heard.

Throughout these pages, you will find a blend of theory and practice woven together with real-world examples, case studies, and reflective prompts designed to ignite insight and provoke critical thinking. This approach honours the complexity of care settings where one size never fits all, and where assessments must be as fluid and responsive as the needs and environments they serve. By exploring diverse risk scenarios and control strategies, we aim to equip you with a versatile toolkit that enhances both your confidence and competence. The inclusion of safe working systems, dynamic risk assessments in emergencies, and person-centred approaches rooted in respect and empowerment ensures you are prepared to meet the everyday challenges and unexpected crises that define the sector.

The legal frameworks that underpin practice in the UK form an essential pillar of this book. Understanding legislation such as the Health and Safety at Work Act 1974 and the standards set by the Care Quality Commission provides not only a roadmap for compliance but also a lens through which to view your professional responsibilities and ethical commitments. These frameworks are not mere regulations; they are the embodiment of societal expectations and protective measures that safeguard the welfare of all stakeholders. Navigating these frameworks does not mean rigid constraint; rather, it invites mindful adherence coupled with thoughtful interpretation to foster environments where care can thrive safely and respectfully.

Beyond compliance and control lies the vital theme of empowerment. Risk assessment is often mistakenly perceived as a barrier to service user independence, yet this book firmly advocates for positive risk-taking as an ethical imperative. Supporting individuals to make informed choices, accepting manageable risks to enhance quality of life, requires skill, sensitivity, and courage. We explore how care providers can champion this balance, maintaining safety without eroding dignity or agency. Person-centred risk assessments are demystified here, emphasising active involvement of service users and collaborative decision-making that honours personal narratives and aspirations.

No single professional or agency can shoulder the responsibility for risk management alone. This work profoundly emphasises the power of multi-agency collaboration and open communication to safeguard well-being and improve outcomes. Whether navigating safeguarding concerns, infection control, or lone working challenges, the interconnectedness of roles and the necessity for transparent, accurate documentation and reporting become apparent. The culture of continuous improvement that the book promotes is one that embraces reflection, responsive adaptation, and shared accountability, creating a workforce increasingly reliable, resilient, and respectful of diversity and complexity.

It is my sincere hope that as you engage with this text, you will find not only knowledge but inspiration; not only protocols but purpose. Risk assessment is often viewed through a lens of problem and prevention, but here it is also portrayed as a catalyst for positive change, a means to champion safety, independence, dignity, and quality in equal measure. The diverse voices of care providers, managers, service users, and regulators converge throughout these pages to illuminate both the challenges and the immense rewards inherent in this vital work.

Whether you are new to health and social care or an experienced professional seeking to deepen your understanding and refine your practice, ***"Mastering Risk Assessment in Health and Social Care: Protecting Life, Improving Care***" is designed to meet you where you are and guide you forward. With practical tools, reflective questions, and real-world scenarios, the book invites you into an ongoing dialogue about risk not as a threat to be feared, but as a reality to be embraced thoughtfully and responsibly.

As you turn these pages, may you feel equipped to make a meaningful difference in the lives of those you serve, and to foster environments rich in safety, respect, and empowerment. Together, through knowledge and compassion, we can elevate the standard of care and transform risk assessment from a daunting obligation into a powerful mechanism for positive, person-centred change.

Welcome to a journey of discovery, reflection, and professional growth. Let us begin.

Introduction to Risk Assessment

Definition of Risk Assessment

In the realm of health and social care, understanding the precise meanings of 'risk' and 'hazard' is foundational to the art and science of risk assessment, serving as the bedrock upon which safe and effective care is built. A hazard, in its essence, can be described as any source or situation that has the potential to cause harm. This might manifest as physical dangers such as wet floors that increase the likelihood of slips and falls, biological threats like infectious agents that jeopardise health through contamination, chemical compounds that can result in poisoning or burns, or even psychological stressors that affect mental well-being. It is critical to recognise that hazards are inherent elements or conditions within environments, processes, or behaviours that could, under specific circumstances, lead to injury, illness, or damage. For instance, a resident's exposure to poorly maintained mobility aids poses a hazard due to the potential for malfunction and harm.

Risk, in contrast, moves beyond the mere presence of these hazards to encompass the probability of an adverse event occurring because of that hazard, as well as the severity of its consequences. It serves as a dynamic measure that reflects the interaction among three key factors: the nature of the hazard, the vulnerability of the exposed person, and the context of exposure. For example, while a wet floor is a hazard, the risk it poses is higher for an elderly resident with limited balance than for a young, agile staff member. Risk, therefore, encompasses both chance and impact, underscoring the variability that makes risk management a nuanced endeavour rather than a static checklist.

The essential distinction between hazard and risk lies in this interplay: hazards are potential threats that are inherently present, whereas risk represents the calculated likelihood that these hazards will translate into actual harm. Appreciating this difference is crucial because the process of risk assessment is not merely to list hazards but to evaluate how these hazards might affect individuals within a given setting, guiding targeted interventions to mitigate chance and consequence effectively. Without this clarity, efforts can become superficial, either over-alarmist or dangerously complacent, neither of which serves the goal of safeguarding health and promoting wellbeing.

Risk assessment, then, emerges as a systematic, structured process designed to identify hazards, analyse and evaluate the associated risks, and implement appropriate control measures to reduce those risks to acceptable levels. This cyclical and ongoing exercise is vital within health and social care environments to ensure the safety of service users, staff, and visitors alike. It encompasses not only physical safety but also the protection of psychological and emotional health, reflecting a holistic understanding of wellbeing. The significance of risk assessment is amplified in care settings, where the vulnerability of individuals due to age, disability, illness, or complex social factors demands thorough scrutiny of potential risks and a thoughtful balance between risk reduction and the promotion of dignity, autonomy, and quality of life.

Beyond its practical function, risk assessment embodies a legal and moral imperative enshrined in the regulatory frameworks and legislation that govern health and social care in the United Kingdom. The Health and Safety at Work Act of 1974 stands as a cornerstone statute, establishing the legal duty of employers to ensure, so far as reasonably practicable, the health, safety, and welfare of all employees and other people affected by their operations. Within this legislative landscape, risk assessments are not optional exercises but mandatory practices integral to compliance. The Act requires that hazards be identified, risks evaluated, and measures taken to manage or eliminate risks effectively. Moreover, specialised regulations like the Management of Health and Safety at Work Regulations 1999 expand upon these duties by compelling employers to carry out suitable and sufficient risk assessments, articulate safety arrangements, and review them regularly.

Complementing these statutes is the oversight of regulatory bodies such as the Care Quality Commission (CQC), which sets and monitors standards for health and social care providers. The CQC's framework consistently emphasises the necessity of effective risk management as a fundamental element of safe, responsive, and well-led services. Their guidance reinforces the principle that risk assessments must be person-centred, involving service users and reflecting individual needs, preferences, and capacities. This approach ensures that risk management does not become a sterilising force that erodes independence but rather supports positive risk-taking as a vehicle for enhancing wellbeing and social inclusion.

The legal and regulatory environment thus creates a mesh of accountability that envelops everyone within care settings, from the macro levels of organisational governance to the frontline practitioners delivering day-to-day care. Employers bear overarching responsibilities to establish, resource, and monitor risk assessment processes, fostering cultures where risk awareness and safety are embedded values. Managers hold critical roles in implementing policies, training staff, and ensuring assessments are comprehensive, current, and accessible. Employees and care providers are entrusted to actively engage with these procedures, recognising hazards, reporting concerns, adhering to control measures, and contributing to continuous risk evaluation. Risk assessors, whether dedicated specialists or practitioners with delegated responsibility, bring expertise to the process, coordinating data collection, analysis, and the crafting of action plans.

Together, these roles create a tapestry of shared accountability that strengthens resilience against harm. In health and social care, the very essence of risk assessment is intertwined with ethical considerations: it demands respect for the dignity and autonomy of service users while safeguarding their safety and that of others. This delicate balance is why risk assessment transcends a mere technical or bureaucratic task, becoming a vital conversation among all stakeholders about values, rights, and responsibilities. Its significance is further underscored by the dynamic nature of care environments, where changing health conditions, diverse needs, and unpredictable scenarios require flexible, responsive risk management that can adapt quickly and thoughtfully.

In summary, risk and hazard are interrelated but distinct concepts that collectively inform the vital activity of risk assessment in health and social care. Identifying hazards shines a light on potential dangers; evaluating risk measures the likelihood and impact of those dangers affecting individuals; and risk assessment synthesises these insights into strategic plans to minimise harm. Within the regulatory framework established by laws such as the Health and Safety at Work Act and standards enforced by the Care Quality Commission, risk assessment is a non-negotiable obligation that ensures safety, promotes positive risk-taking, and upholds the dignity and empowerment of those receiving and providing care. The ongoing engagement and shared responsibilities among employers, managers, practitioners, and service users embed risk assessment as a cornerstone of quality and compassionate care, illustrating its profound significance beyond paperwork into the heart of health and social care delivery.

Legal and Regulatory Framework

In the intricate and ever-evolving landscape of health and social care, the legal and regulatory framework forms the backbone of safety, accountability, and a culture in which risk management is not merely a best practice but a legal obligation. Understanding this framework is essential not only for compliance but also for truly safeguarding the dignity and well-being of service users while protecting care providers themselves. At the heart of this legal tapestry lies the Health and

Safety at Work Act 1974 (HSWA), a seminal piece of legislation that has shaped the approach to risk management across all sectors, including health and social care. The Act establishes a comprehensive duty of care that employers owe to their employees and, by extension, to those who might be affected by their undertaking, namely, service users, visitors, and the wider public. This duty imposes an unequivocal responsibility on all employers to ensure, as far as reasonably practicable, the health, safety, and welfare of their staff at work, thereby setting the foundational standard that cascades down through various regulations and guidance.

The HSWA is distinctive not by prescribing detailed safety measures but by establishing a broad, adaptive framework that requires organisations to actively assess and manage risks. This breadth is intentional; it ensures that, rather than being bound to rigid protocols that might overlook the nuances of individual care settings, providers must develop risk assessments and control measures tailored to their unique environments, needs, and challenges. This Act is the legal bedrock upon which other regulations and standards are constructed, and its influence is far-reaching. Importantly, it also underscores employees' rights by mandating their cooperation with employers in health and safety arrangements and by prohibiting interference with safety equipment, reinforcing a culture of shared responsibility.

Complementing the HSWA are more specific regulations that provide structured detail on how risk should be managed and controlled. The Management of Health and Safety at Work Regulations 1999 (MHSWR) is a pivotal example. This set of regulations amplifies the HSWA by requiring employers to conduct appropriate and timely risk assessments that identify hazards and evaluate risks to health and safety for both employees and those affected by their work activities. The MHSWR explicitly requires that these risk assessments be regularly reviewed and documented when five or more employees are involved, thereby ensuring sustained vigilance. What makes the MHSWR particularly influential in health and social care is its insistence on establishing effective arrangements to manage health and safety, including planning, organisation, control, monitoring, and review. The regulations require a clear designation of health and safety responsibilities within the organisation, highlighting that management is not merely about policy but about action, leadership, and accountability.

Central figures in this regulatory landscape are the employers and managers who must not only comprehend these requirements but also translate them into operational practices. They are required to allocate sufficient resources, time, personnel, training, and funding to implement effective risk management systems. Their roles necessitate a continuous dialogue with front-line care providers to gain insights from direct experience, thereby moulding risk assessments that are realistic, applicable, and person-centred. Simultaneously, employees themselves are entrusted with the duty to engage proactively, following established controls, reporting hazards, and contributing their knowledge toward refining safety measures. These dual dynamics foster an environment where risk assessment is a collaborative and iterative process, reflecting the fluid and often unpredictable nature of health and social care settings.

Parallel to these legislative acts are the standards established by regulatory bodies that oversee and inspect the provision of care to uphold quality and safety. In the United Kingdom, the Care Quality Commission (CQC) serves as the principal regulator for health and social care services, enforcing compliance through a comprehensive framework of standards. The CQC's Fundamental Standards, integral to its inspection regime, directly encapsulate expectations around risk management, safeguarding, and the provision of safe care and treatment. These standards mandate that providers must systematically assess risks, implement adequate measures to mitigate them, and continuously review outcomes to foster improvement. The CQC requires clear evidence that risk assessments are tailored for individual service users, respecting their rights to dignity and autonomy while ensuring their safety. This underscores a progressive approach that balances risk reduction with empowerment, a key paradigm shift in care delivery.

The impact of the CQC's role is profound, as it extends beyond mere compliance checks to foster a culture of openness, learning, and accountability. Providers are expected to maintain accurate records of risk assessments and associated actions, report incidents, including 'near misses,' and participate in multi-agency safeguarding collaborations when necessary. Through public reporting and transparency, the CQC not only holds providers to account but also supports service users and their families in making informed decisions about care. Their approach mirrors contemporary understandings that risk management must be transparent, evidence-based, and subject to continuous scrutiny and enhancement.

Beyond the central pillars of HSWA, MHSWR, and CQC standards, the regulatory framework encompasses a constellation of related legislation and guidance, each contributing essential facets to the overall risk management ecosystem. For example, the Reporting of Injuries, Diseases and

Dangerous Occurrences Regulations (RIDDOR) 2013 require the notification of specified work-related incidents, thereby ensuring that serious events or patterns of harm are appropriately escalated and investigated. This legal duty to report fosters a systemic approach to learning from adverse events and preventing recurrence.

Similarly, the Control of Substances Hazardous to Health (COSHH) Regulations 2002 impose a duty to assess and mitigate risks related to exposure to toxic substances, a critical concern in settings where chemicals, cleaning agents, and medicines are handled routinely. These regulations require that risks be identified, control measures be implemented, and staff be trained accordingly, thereby integrating chemical safety into broader health and safety practices. The Personal Protective Equipment at Work Regulations 1992 further complement these by stipulating when and how protective gear must be provided and used, emphasising that risk control is not only about policy but practical, everyday protections.

In the context of the Mental Capacity Act 2005 and the associated Deprivation of Liberty Safeguards (DoLS), legal imperatives also shape how risk assessments must respect the autonomy and rights of individuals who may lack capacity. The balancing act here is delicate; safeguarding individuals without unnecessarily restricting their freedoms requires careful, legally informed risk assessment and documentation. Failure to meet these standards can result in both legal consequences and harm to service users, underscoring the critical nature of comprehensive knowledge of relevant laws and their ethical implications.

The convergence of these laws and regulations creates a complex but coherent legal framework that governs how risk is identified, assessed, controlled, documented, and reviewed within health and social care. This framework underscores the necessity of embedding a robust risk culture within organisations, one that integrates legal requirements with professional judgment, person-centred care, and continuous learning. The roles and responsibilities within this framework are distributed deliberately, with employers and managers bearing ultimate accountability, tasked with establishing systems and allocating resources; employees must exercise diligence and cooperation; professional assessors bring expertise; and regulatory agencies monitor and enforce standards.

At the operational level, this means that risk assessments cannot be viewed as static, isolated documents but rather dynamic processes embedded in organisational practice and culture. They are living tools for anticipating hazards, managing uncertainty, and protecting all involved. This approach requires that trained staff be equipped not only with the technical skills to identify risks but also with a clear understanding of their legal obligations and the ethical dimensions underpinning their work. Training and education, therefore, become pivotal elements, ensuring that knowledge of legislation is translated into practice that safeguards rights, promotes dignity, and facilitates positive risk-taking, a crucial concept in contemporary care aimed at enhancing independence rather than imposing undue restriction.

Moreover, accountability mechanisms embedded within the legal and regulatory framework are backed by sanctions and enforcement powers. Regulatory agencies like the CQC can issue warnings, impose conditions on registration, or even prosecute providers who fail to meet required standards. Enforcement notices compel remedial action, and prosecutions under HSWA or related laws carry penalties ranging from fines to imprisonment. These responses serve as stark reminders of the serious implications of neglecting risk management and demonstrate the state's commitment to upholding public safety and trust.

Integral to these enforcement processes is the requirement for meticulous documentation. Legal compliance is inseparable from accurate recording of risk assessments, control measures, training, incidents, and communications. Well-maintained records provide evidence of due diligence, facilitate audits and inspections, and form the basis for continuous improvement. They also serve as critical tools in multi-agency collaboration, enabling seamless information sharing vital to safeguarding vulnerable individuals.

The regulatory framework thus guides organisations toward embedding risk assessment not as a bureaucratic requirement but as a living, evolving practice that protects lives, supports rights, and enhances quality of care. It demands that risk assessment be integrated within governance structures, quality assurance, staff supervision, and policy development. Care providers must design risk management systems that are responsive to changing environments, such as emerging health threats or shifting service-user needs, to ensure resilience and adaptability.

In summary, the legal and regulatory framework encompassing the Health and Safety at Work Act 1974, the Management of Health and Safety at Work Regulations 1999, the CQC Fundamental Standards, and complementary legislation forms a comprehensive web that mandates and shapes risk assessment in health and social care. It sets clear duties and responsibilities for all stakeholders while promoting a culture of safety, learning, and respect. Understanding and operationalising this framework is indispensable for care providers seeking to deliver safe, effective, and dignified care. It empowers them to navigate the complex challenges of their environments confidently and to make decisions that balance safety with empowerment, in full alignment with statutory obligations and ethical imperatives. Through this legal lens, risk assessment emerges not as a constraint but as a powerful enabler of high-quality care and positive outcomes for all involved.

Roles and Responsibilities

In the complex and dynamic environment of health and social care, the effective management of risk hinges largely upon a clear understanding of roles and responsibilities across all levels of the workforce. Risk assessment is not the task of a single individual: it is an integrated process requiring the dedicated engagement of employers, employees, managers, and specialist risk assessors alike. Each of these roles carries distinct yet interconnected duties that, when performed collaboratively and conscientiously, serve to create safer, more supportive environments for both service users and care providers. It is within this collective dedication that risk assessment transcends paperwork and protocol, becoming a living practice that protects dignity, encourages positive risk-taking, and ensures regulatory compliance.

Employers bear the overarching responsibility for establishing and maintaining a safe working and care environment. This duty encompasses a broad spectrum of actions, beginning with the establishment of comprehensive risk management policies that align with national legislation, such as the Health and Safety at Work Act 1974, and with regulations set by the Care Quality Commission (CQC). Employers are obligated to provide the necessary resources for risk assessment processes, ensuring that staff receive adequate training, supervision, and support to recognise, report, and mitigate hazards effectively. Beyond supplying resources, employers must foster a workplace culture where safety and openness are prioritised and where continuous improvement mechanisms are in place for reviewing risk practices systematically. This includes facilitating access to relevant information and updated guidelines, and establishing clear channels for communication and feedback across all levels of personnel.

The duty of employers extends to the provision and maintenance of safe work systems and environments. This means ensuring that the physical premises, equipment, and procedural protocols do not pose undue risks to anyone in the care setting. Employers must also act decisively to eliminate or reduce identified risks, which may involve investing in updated technologies, redesigning workflows, or implementing safer alternatives to hazardous substances or methods. Importantly, employers must ensure legal compliance by completing and maintaining documented risk assessments as mandatory evidence of due diligence. They retain accountability not only for meeting statutory requirements but also for encouraging and enabling their workforce to engage positively with risk, recognising that excessive risk aversion can detract from the independence and well-being of service users.

Meanwhile, employees at all levels hold pivotal responsibilities in operationalising risk management strategies. Care workers, support staff, and other frontline employees are required to actively identify hazards in their daily work environment and contribute to risk assessments from their frontline perspective. They must uphold safe working practices meticulously and adhere strictly to the control measures established by their employer. Employees are expected to remain vigilant and proactive, reporting potential risks, near misses, or breaches of safety procedures promptly through established channels. In doing so, they help to mitigate hazards before they can result in harm. This duty to report extends to embracing a transparent and open approach in raising concerns, which is vital in nurturing a risk-aware culture.

Employees are also responsible for maintaining their competency through continuous professional development, particularly as safety protocols and risk factors evolve with changes in care delivery models and emerging public health challenges. Participation in training sessions and refreshers ensures that employees can recognise subtle or emergent risks and respond appropriately. In settings where complex and unpredictable situations frequently arise, such as mental health, community care, or domiciliary settings, employees' capacity to dynamically perform risk assessments is crucial. Their input is especially significant in person-centred risk assessments where the preferences, needs, and autonomy of service users must be respected alongside safety imperatives. Hence, staff members must exercise professional judgment with resilience, balancing safety with empowerment.

Managers serve as the critical nexus between the strategic oversight provided by employers and the operational delivery carried out by employees. They have multifaceted responsibilities that extend beyond personal adherence to safety standards. Managers are tasked with coordinating the risk assessment process across their teams and ensuring that all identified risks are systematically evaluated, documented, and addressed with appropriate control measures. This involves scheduling and overseeing regular workplace inspections and audits, investigating incidents or accidents to identify causative factors, and applying lessons learned to policy and practice improvements. Managers must champion embedding risk management within everyday organisational culture, encouraging their teams to approach risk as an integral element of care rather than an obstructive afterthought.

In fulfilling their role, managers must ensure that risk assessments and resulting action plans are realistic, measurable, and monitored for efficacy over time. They act as conduits for communication between frontline staff and senior leadership, providing feedback loops that inform resource allocation, training needs, and procedural adjustments. A manager's ability to balance compliance demands with the care philosophy of promoting independence requires nuanced judgment, especially when dealing with risk-averse tendencies from within the team or from external regulators. Holding responsibility for ensuring accountability means managers must also support and guide staff through complex ethical dilemmas that arise during risk assessment processes, in safeguarding decisions, or when service users' choices may increase their vulnerability.

In many organisations, designated risk assessors or health and safety specialists provide additional focused expertise. These individuals often bring advanced knowledge of legislative requirements, industry best practices, and risk management theories. Their role is to support the broader team by crafting comprehensive risk assessment frameworks, advising on technical matters such as infection control, hazardous materials handling, and emergency preparedness. In complex cases such as infection outbreaks, abuse allegations, or when service users have multiple co-morbidities, risk assessors contribute expert evaluation, assisting managers and care providers in tailoring individualised care plans that appropriately balance risk with autonomy. They may also facilitate training sessions dedicated specifically to risk management competencies and advise on record-keeping and reporting protocols essential for audit trails and legal compliance.

While employers, employees, managers, and risk assessors each hold discrete responsibilities, the very nature of health and social care demands fluid collaboration. For instance, an employee reporting a risk must have confidence in their manager's responsiveness, just as a manager relies on accurate input from frontline staff and guidance from health and safety experts to adjust practices effectively. Similarly, employers set the tone and resources upon which this cooperative framework depends, making the interdependence among roles a fundamental principle in risk management.

Importantly, legal and regulatory frameworks underpin these roles with statutory clarity while also emphasising the principle of 'reasonableness', requiring all practical steps within capacity to ensure safety. The Health and Safety at Work Act 1974 specifically mandates that employers "so far as is reasonably practicable" safeguard the health, safety, and welfare of employees and others affected by their operations. This phrase calls for a balanced approach rather than unattainable perfection, reinforcing the need for everyone in the organisation to engage responsibly in risk management. The CQC further enforces these duties by inspecting and rating services on safety and governance aspects, holding employers and managers to account for compliance with safeguarding, infection control, medication safety, and other risk-related domains.

Through such regulatory oversight, roles and responsibilities assume enforceability, reminding all stakeholders that risk management is not optional but an essential component of care quality and legal duty. Employers risk prosecution and financial penalties for negligence, managers may face disciplinary action for failures in oversight, and employees could be held accountable if grossly negligent. Conversely, demonstrating strict adherence to roles within risk assessment processes provides a protective shield for both the care organisation and its individuals against liability and reputational damage.

At a deeper level, the ethical dimension of roles and responsibilities cannot be overstated. Every duty carried by employers, managers, employees, and risk assessors is in service of protecting vulnerable individuals while respecting their rights and dignity. The relational aspects of care require that risk management is never exclusively about safety in isolation but is tightly woven with principles of autonomy, empowerment, and compassion. Care providers must recognise that facilitating positive risk-taking, enabling service users to engage in meaningful activities that carry some level of risk, is essential to sustaining quality of life and personal growth. This perspective demands that roles not only execute technical risk assessment tasks but also negotiate complex interpersonal dynamics, advocate for service users' voices, and challenge risk-averse cultures when necessary.

In practical terms, this means employers must invest in creating supportive environments in which staff feel psychologically safe raising concerns or making recommendations. Managers must embody leadership that respects diverse risk tolerances, provide supervision that encourages reflective practice, and mediate tensions between safety policies and service users' wishes. Employees must practice skilled communication, empathy, and professional judgement in risk conversations with service users, families, and colleagues. Risk assessors, in their advisory capacity, must promote ethical frameworks that integrate legal compliance with human rights and social justice considerations.

The accountability embedded within these roles is reinforced by documentation and reporting standards, which serve not only as records of compliance but as tools for learning and transparency. A clear definition of roles facilitates responsibility-sharing, ensuring that no aspect of risk is overlooked and that corrective actions are distributed appropriately. In essence, the roles and responsibilities create a web of interlinked duties where each actor's contribution is vital. Without employers' vision and commitment, managers' coordination, employees' diligence, and risk assessors' expertise, the risk assessment process would falter.

Ultimately, the dynamic interaction of these roles sustains a culture of safety and continuous improvement. As health and social care environments evolve with changing demographics, emerging technologies, and shifting policy landscapes, these roles adapt, always revolving around the core imperative to protect and empower. Together, they form the backbone of risk assessment practices that not only comply with legal mandates but also elevate standards of care, ensuring that services remain responsive, ethical, and resilient in the face of complexity.

Identifying Hazards

Types of Hazards in Health and Social Care

Within the intricate tapestry of health and social care, hazards permeate nearly every aspect of daily operations, posing ongoing challenges to the safety and well-being of both service users and care providers. Recognising the multifaceted nature of these hazards is not merely an academic exercise but a vital professional skill that underpins effective risk assessment and management. The diverse environments in which care is delivered, from bustling hospitals and intimate community settings to residential homes and specialised day centres, each carry unique exposures to risks, making the vigilant identification and understanding of hazard types an indispensable part of safeguarding. To embark on this journey of understanding, it is essential to traverse the broad terrain of hazard categories: physical, biological, chemical, environmental, and psychological, each embodying distinct dangers yet often interlacing, compounding the complexities caregivers face.

Physical hazards constitute one of the most immediate and visible threats in health and social care settings. These hazards encompass any physical environment or conditions that may cause bodily harm. Commonly, these include slips, trips, and falls, which sit among the leading causes of injury in care facilities. Floors left wet after cleaning without timely signage, uneven surfaces, or cluttered walkways can quickly turn routine movements into perilous endeavours. For instance, a service user with limited mobility may face heightened risks from a misplaced chair or an unsecured rug, illustrating how familiar domestic items can transform into hazards. Similarly, moving and handling patients or equipment exposes care providers to musculoskeletal injuries due to awkward postures, heavy lifting, or repetitive strain, particularly where adequate training or assistive devices are lacking. Equipment itself, such as malfunctioning wheelchairs, walkers, or hoists, can become physical hazards when not properly maintained, underscoring how the very tools designed to assist can sometimes endanger. In addition, electrical hazards arise from faulty wiring or damaged plugs and sockets, potentially leading to shocks or fire. Other physical risks include exposure to radiation, such as that used in diagnostic procedures like X-rays, where protective measures must be rigorously observed. The tangible nature of physical hazards and their predictability through routine inspections and hazard spotting make them primary targets for preventive efforts.

Parallel to physical hazards, biological hazards add an invisible yet equally potent threat within health and social care environments. These hazards arise from exposure to harmful microorganisms, viruses, parasites, or bodily fluids, factors that could precipitate infections, disease outbreaks, or severe health complications. The vulnerability of service users, often with compromised immune systems or chronic conditions, magnifies the peril posed by such biological agents. Common examples include bloodborne pathogens such as HIV or hepatitis B and C, which health professionals face particularly when handling needles or sharp instruments. Moreover, respiratory illnesses caused by airborne pathogens such as influenza and tuberculosis demonstrate how easily infections spread in enclosed spaces where care is provided. The presence of contaminated surfaces, improperly disposed of clinical waste, or inadequate hand hygiene further escalates the biological risk, emphasising the critical role of infection control measures, including the use of personal protective equipment (PPE) and stringent cleaning protocols. Beyond direct human pathogens, biological hazards extend to exposure to mould, fungi, or pests, often exacerbated by poor environmental maintenance, which can trigger allergic reactions or respiratory difficulties. Each of these invisible hazards demands constant vigilance, exacting standards, and rapid response strategies to protect vulnerable populations and staff alike.

Chemical hazards, often underestimated in health and social care settings, emerge from exposure to substances that can be toxic, corrosive, flammable, or irritant. These include a vast array of cleaning agents, disinfectants, medications, and laboratory reagents that caregivers regularly handle. Despite their routine use, careless handling or improper storage can lead to significant health risks, including skin burns, respiratory problems, poisoning, or chemical burns. For example, concentrated bleach solutions or sanitising solvents can cause respiratory irritation or dermatitis if contact precautions are neglected. Medication errors involving overdose or accidental ingestion by service users may introduce chemical hazards with dire consequences. Moreover, hazardous substances can include radiopharmaceuticals or cytotoxic drugs used in cancer therapies, requiring highly skilled handling and specific safety protocols. The storage of chemicals poses its own challenges: incompatible substances kept adjacent could react dangerously, leading to fires or the release of harmful gases. Awareness of Safety Data Sheets (SDS) is critical for staff to comprehend the properties of chemicals they encounter, ensuring proper labelling, handling, and emergency response. Ultimately, the chemical hazard domain demands a culture of respect toward potentially dangerous substances, underpinned by comprehensive training and meticulous adherence to control measures.

The environmental category of hazards contextualises the physical surroundings that envelop health and social care settings, broadening the viewpoint beyond immediate hazards to encompass factors that influence safety and operational effectiveness on a grander scale. Elements such as poor ventilation, inadequate lighting, extreme temperatures, and noise pollution can undermine both mental and physical health if left unaddressed. For instance, dimly lit corridors may obscure obstacles, increasing the risk of physical hazards, while poor air circulation fosters an environment conducive to infections or exacerbates respiratory conditions. Temperature extremes, either excessive heat or cold, can harm service users, especially those with frail health or sensory impairments, causing dehydration, hypothermia, or heat stroke. Noise, often an overlooked hazard, can elevate stress levels for both staff and service users, disrupt communication critical to safe care, and contribute to fatigue or burnout. Moreover, structural hazards affecting building integrity, such as faulty stair rails, unstable flooring, or inadequate fire exits, pose lurking dangers whose consequences could be catastrophic during emergencies. Environmental hazards also extend outdoors, where weather conditions and uneven grounds can heighten risks during community visits or garden activities. Recognising these multifactorial, pervasive threats obliges services to embed environmental assessments into their routine safety audits and foster a responsive approach to correcting and improving the care milieu.

Psychological hazards, though less tangible than physical risks, wield profound influence over well-being and care delivery, affecting service users and care providers alike. Stress, anxiety, burnout, workplace violence, harassment, and moral distress constitute various facets of psychological hazards that can erode professional effectiveness, compromise safety, and diminish service quality. For care providers, managing the emotional toll of supporting vulnerable individuals, facing high workloads, or encountering aggressive behaviour demands robust resilience and organisational support. Unmanaged psychological hazards increase absenteeism and staff turnover, which ripple out to affect continuity and stability for service users. For those receiving care, psychological hazards may include feelings of isolation, loss of autonomy, fear, or the trauma of abuse or neglect, highlighting a critical ethical and safeguarding dimension. The mental health of service users can be acutely sensitive to environment and interpersonal dynamics, with psychological hazards often manifesting through subtle behavioural changes or deteriorating engagement. Identifying and responding to these hazards demands sensitive observation skills, open communication channels, and measures such as counselling support, conflict-resolution training, and fostering positive workplace cultures. Importantly, psychological hazards closely intersect with physical safety, as stress and fatigue impair attention and judgment, potentially precipitating accidents or errors. An acknowledgement of psychological risks broadens the notion of hazard beyond the physical, affirming the humanity at the heart of care.

Proactive hazard identification in health and social care settings relies not only on understanding these broad categories but equally on deploying systematic tools and techniques that bridge theory and practice. Workplace inspections remain a foundational approach, in which trained personnel conduct detailed observations of the physical environment, equipment, and work processes to identify potential hazards. Such inspections, when performed regularly and methodically, illuminate issues before they escalate, enabling timely interventions and reinforcing a culture of vigilance. Beyond scheduled audits, reactive incident reporting systems serve as critical feedback loops, capturing data on near misses, accidents, or unsafe practices. These reports offer rich insights, often revealing hazards not immediately apparent during inspections, and empower staff to actively participate in safety improvement by sharing frontline experiences. Encouraging a blame-free reporting environment is essential to ensure openness and continual hazard detection. Similarly, informal feedback mechanisms, including staff meetings, suggestion boxes, or one-on-one supervision sessions, provide avenues to surface concerns and innovative ideas for hazard mitigation. For example, a care worker might highlight that a particular route used for patient transfers becomes slippery during rainy weather, prompting preventive action. Observational techniques, such as shadowing staff during their daily routines or engaging with service users, help uncover dynamic hazards that emerge under fluctuating conditions, for instance, during emergencies or behavioural crises. Integrating technology, such as environmental sensors or digital monitoring tools, increasingly complements traditional methods, offering real-time alerts on temperature fluctuations or chemical exposures.

The interplay of these tools fosters a layered, responsive hazard identification strategy essential for the fluid contexts encountered in health and social care. Importantly, effective hazard recognition is not an endpoint but a continuum that must adapt to evolving challenges, organisational changes, and emerging care models. Building competencies in hazard identification at all levels, from frontline care providers to management and regulatory bodies, ensures a shared-responsibility ethos that is pivotal to safeguarding environments. Furthermore, involving service users themselves in identifying hazards respects their lived experiences and rights, illuminates risks that are invisible to professionals, and enhances person-centred care. This inclusive approach nurtures empowerment and aligns safety objectives with the dignity and independence that underpin quality care. Ultimately, embracing the breadth of hazard types and the multifaceted strategy for their detection equips health and social care practitioners with the foresight and tools necessary to navigate and mitigate the complex landscape of risk, turning potential threats into managed, meaningful opportunities for improvement and compassionate safety.

Methods of Identifying Hazards

Recognising hazards in health and social care settings is a pivotal first step to ensuring the safety and well-being of both service users and care providers. Hazards in such environments can manifest in numerous forms, physical, biological, chemical, environmental, and psychological, each posing unique risks that demand keen awareness and responsive identification techniques. The process of identifying these hazards must be systematic and ongoing, rooted not only in regulatory compliance but in fostering a proactive safety culture that anticipates potential threats before they materialise into harm. The practical approaches to hazard identification are manifold, each offering valuable insights and complementary perspectives that, when combined, create a robust shield against the occurrence of risk.

One of the most foundational methods employed in hazard identification is the workplace inspection. This approach involves systematic, planned surveys of the care environment, designed to detect potential risks within the physical settings and working practices. Inspections can be routine or intermittent, often following a schedule that aligns with organisational policies or regulatory recommendations. The effectiveness of workplace inspections rests on their thoroughness and the expertise of those conducting them. Skilled inspectors, who possess a deep understanding of health and social care contexts, can uncover hidden or latent hazards that might escape casual observation. These inspections extend beyond the obvious physical hazards, such as slippery floors or faulty equipment. They delve into subtler threats such as inadequate lighting that could impair vision and increase the likelihood of accidents, spatial layouts that risk overcrowding and impede emergency evacuation, or the presence of biohazards in poorly maintained sanitation facilities.

The process is enhanced by comprehensive checklists tailored to the specific demands of health and social care environments. These checklists serve as systematic guides to ensure no area or potential risk source is overlooked. They are dynamic tools, evolving alongside emerging knowledge about risks and incorporating feedback from previous inspections and incident analyses. Workplace inspections promote direct engagement with the environment and foster a culture of vigilance. They often involve multidisciplinary teams, including care providers, safety officers, and managers, pooling observational skills and expertise. The collaborative nature of inspections not only expedites hazard detection but also strengthens shared ownership of safety responsibilities.

In addition to planned inspections, spontaneous walkthroughs or informal observations provide invaluable opportunities for real-time hazard identification. These observations, when made routinely by staff in their work, empower every individual to act as a sentry for safety. Staff members, frequently immersed in day-to-day care delivery, are uniquely positioned to notice emerging hazards arising from evolving care dynamics, equipment wear and tear, or environmental changes. Encouraging open lines of communication so that staff feel comfortable reporting potential hazards as they arise is essential. It transforms hazard identification from a formal task into an ingrained behavioural norm permeating workplace culture.

Complementing observational strategies are the systematic reviews of accident and incident reports. These documentation-based approaches offer rich, data-driven insights into hazard patterns and their consequences. Each report represents a narrative of what went wrong, where, when, and possibly why, revealing vulnerabilities within the care system. By analysing these reports collectively, organisations can identify recurring themes and underlying conditions that precipitate hazards. For example, repeated incidents involving manual handling injuries may indicate deficiencies in training, inadequate equipment, or flawed care practices, highlighting physical risks in the workplace. These insights trigger focused hazard-identification efforts that target root causes rather than superficial fixes.

Moreover, accident reports help illuminate less visible hazards, such as psychological stressors that contribute to errors or behavioural risks in service users that jeopardise safety. The systematic use of incident reporting is a cornerstone of reactive hazard identification, transforming adverse events into learning opportunities that pre-empt future harm. It requires a non-punitive, supportive reporting culture in which staff are motivated to report without fear of blame, ensuring that comprehensive and candid information is available for review.

Feedback mechanisms form another crucial conduit for hazard identification, involving direct inputs from staff, service users, and visitors. These feedback channels may take various forms, including surveys, suggestion boxes, structured interviews, focus groups, or informal conversations. The value of feedback lies in its co-creative nature, offering lived-experience perspectives that may elude technical assessments or inspection protocols. For instance, a service user who feels anxious about a particular area of the facility might reveal psychological hazards stemming from environmental design or interpersonal dynamics. Staff may highlight systemic issues that contribute to hazards, such as insufficient staffing levels that increase stress and the likelihood of mistakes. Feedback loops are instrumental in capturing the subtleties of psychosocial risks and emerging hazards related to changes in care demands or organisational culture.

A sophisticated feedback approach integrates formalised forums in which dialogue among care teams, managers, and service users can unearth collective insights into potentially hazardous conditions. Such engagement fosters trust, transparency, and mutual accountability, further embedding safety vigilance into everyday practice. It shifts hazard identification from isolated observation to an evolving conversation that reflects the complex realities of health and social care environments.

Observation also extends into the use of technology-assisted monitoring systems, increasingly adopted to complement human vigilance. Video surveillance, sensor technology, and electronic health records can provide valuable data for dynamically identifying hazards. For example, motion sensors may alert to falls or unusual movements among service users, while electronic records can track medication errors or exposure to infectious agents. However, these tools are most effective when integrated thoughtfully into a broader system of human observation, analysis, and communication, ensuring that the data they generate trigger appropriate responses and further investigation.

Each category of hazard, whether physical, biological, chemical, environmental, or psychological, presents unique challenges that influence the choice and efficacy of identification methods. Physical hazards, such as unsafe equipment or poor ergonomics, can often be detected through diligent inspections and staff observations. Biological hazards, including exposure to pathogens or contaminated materials, require vigilance through infection-control audits and incident reports related to illness or contamination. Chemical hazards, often involving cleaning agents or medications, require inspection of storage and usage protocols, as well as feedback from staff on handling difficulties or breaches. Environmental hazards may arise from factors such as inadequate heating or ventilation, or from external conditions that affect indoor safety, necessitating environmental assessments paired with user feedback on comfort and perceived risk. Psychological hazards such as stress, bullying, or service user aggression are less tangible but potentially devastating, identified primarily through open communication channels, incident reports of aggression or distress, and structured staff support systems.

The synergistic application of these varied approaches ensures a comprehensive identification of hazards. Relying solely on one method risks overlooking subtle or emerging threats. Workplace inspections might miss psychological stressors; incident reports may capture hazards only after harm has occurred; feedback might vary depending on individual willingness and perception. The integration of inspections, reporting, observation, and feedback forms a multi-layered safety net, constantly scanned and refined to maintain a vigilant stance against risk.

Furthermore, the dynamism inherent in health and social care settings, where every day may present new challenges, varied service user needs, and fast-changing environments, necessitates that hazard identification methods are flexible and adaptable. Practices such as dynamic risk assessments, which involve ongoing hazard recognition tied to immediate changes in circumstances, underscore the importance of equipping staff with observational and reporting skills that transcend formal procedures. In such fluid contexts, the ability to recognise hazards in real time, through vigilant observation and swift communication, becomes indispensable.

Effective hazard identification methods also demand appropriate training and cultural reinforcement. Staff must be educated not only on what to look for but why it matters and how to communicate findings constructively. Training programs that incorporate role-playing, scenario analysis, and reflective practice foster a deeper appreciation of hazard diversity and the nuances of detection. Equally, leadership plays a vital role in setting expectations, modelling risk-aware behaviours, and responding effectively to identified hazards. When leaders demonstrate commitment to thorough inspection cycles, value incident reporting, seek broad feedback, and encourage observational contributions, a culture of proactive hazard detection flourishes.

Underlying all practical approaches is the philosophical recognition that hazard identification is not a one-off activity but a continuous commitment. The complex matrix of risk factors in health and social care requires organisations to embed identification strategies in their operational DNA. Only by doing so can they move from reactive firefighting towards anticipatory risk management, protecting those they serve and those who serve with vigilance, empathy, and professionalism.

In conclusion, methods of identifying hazards in health and social care settings encompass a diverse toolkit. Workplace inspections offer structured, systematic scrutiny of physical environments; accident and incident reports provide data-driven reflections on past events; feedback mechanisms bring lived experiences into the spotlight of hazards; while staff observations inject real-time, dynamic recognition of emerging risks. Each method is indispensable, contributing distinct insights that collectively illuminate the full spectrum of hazards threatening safety and well-being. Implementing these methods with rigour, sensitivity, and collaboration equips care providers to anticipate, detect, and manage risks effectively, laying the groundwork for safer, more responsive, and person-centred care environments.

Hazard Identification Case Studies

Within the intricate and often unpredictable settings of health and social care, hazard identification is not merely a procedural step but the foundation upon which safe and effective care hinges. The realities of care environments reveal that hazards come in numerous guises, some overt, striking with conspicuous impact, while others lurk subtly beneath routine operations, almost invisible unless one knows precisely where and how to look. The following case studies provide vivid examples from real-world contexts, illuminating how a deep understanding of various hazard types, combined with practical tools, transforms hazard identification from a theoretical concept into an active, lifesaving skill.

Consider first a community care facility where a new care assistant had recently joined the team. Within her initial weeks, she noticed a frequent slip hazard near the medication administration room. The floor seemed clean, but was often damp due to condensation forming from an ill-maintained air conditioning system. This physical hazard, a wet floor in a high-traffic area, might remain unnoticed without the fresh eyes and observational diligence of a newcomer. The assistant's awareness led to a formal hazard report, which triggered an immediate inspection and repair of the ventilation system. Here, hazard identification emerged from an informal observation and was supported by the established incident reporting mechanism. This case exemplifies how physical hazards such as slips, trips, and falls can often be embedded within the environment in unexpected ways, requiring continuous vigilance and a culture that encourages raising concerns without hesitation.

Shifting focus to a nursing home, a biological hazard posed an insidious threat. An outbreak of norovirus swiftly spread among residents, exposing weaknesses in infection control practices.

Investigation revealed that while staff were diligent with hand hygiene, shared equipment, such as blood pressure cuffs, was not always cleaned between uses. The identification of this biological hazard arose from a combination of clinical observations, meticulous symptom tracking, and feedback from frontline staff who noticed clusters of symptoms occurring after shift changes. These insights prompted a revision of cleaning protocols and staff retraining. This case underscores the complexity of biological hazards; they live not only in the pathogens themselves but in the small, often overlooked practices that facilitate their spread. Effective hazard detection here required a multi-layered approach: clinical vigilance, ongoing communication channels, and a responsive system for gathering and acting on frontline feedback.

In a mental health facility, chemical hazards presented a less conventional but equally significant challenge. Staff members experienced repeated headaches and nausea, initially dismissed as stress-related. Upon closer inspection, it became evident that a nightly cleaning product contained potent volatile organic compounds (VOCs) that were released into poorly ventilated corridors. This environmental chemical hazard had been overlooked due to the ubiquity and familiarity of cleaning procedures. Staff observations and health complaints, collated through informal conversations and formal health surveillance, were instrumental in exposing the risk. The subsequent substitution of the cleaning product with a less harmful alternative, along with enhanced ventilation protocols, markedly improved staff well-being and demonstrated a proactive response to chemical hazards. This scenario highlights that chemical hazards are not confined to laboratory settings but can permeate everyday routines, necessitating ongoing education and attention to the substances introduced into care environments.

Environmental hazards often intersect with physical risks but can have broader implications, as illustrated by a day care centre located near a busy main road. Staff and management wrestled with the challenge of outdoor spaces where children's play areas bordered fast-moving traffic. The primary hazard was the risk of accidentally bolting into the street, an ever-present danger amplified by the surrounding environment. Hazard identification here involved not just a visual inspection but also risk mapping and consultation with service users and their families, who provided invaluable insight into daily practices and vulnerabilities. Staff also employed dynamic observations during different times of the day, noting how varying light conditions and traffic flow patterns influenced risk levels. Consequently, the centre implemented physical controls such as high fencing, secure gates, and staff role rotations to improve supervision during peak traffic hours. This example illustrates environmental hazards as complex phenomena woven into the physical site and social context, demanding innovative and inclusive approaches to their identification and management.

Psychological hazards, though less tangible, can exert profound effects on both service users and care providers. At a residential care unit, rising reports of staff burnout and stress-related absenteeism prompted an in-depth review. Psychological risk factors such as excessive workload, poor communication, and insufficient support systems were identified as key contributors. The hazard identification process here was nuanced: it involved confidential staff surveys, peer discussions facilitated by managers, and reflective practice sessions. These tools revealed underlying pressures that might otherwise have remained hidden beneath surface-level routines. The facility responded with adjustments to staffing levels, the introduction of regular supervisory meetings, and access to counselling services. The outcome was not only improved staff well-being but a noticeable uplift in morale and care quality. This case eloquently demonstrates that psychological hazards require sensitive, often indirect strategies for discovery, and a readiness to listen, reflect, and respond to human factors as legitimate hazards that demand attention equal to that of their physical or biological counterparts.

What threads these case studies together is not only the varied nature of hazards but the critical role of proactive and comprehensive identification methodologies. Workplace inspections, often perceived as routine box-ticking exercises, revealed themselves to be potent tools when thoughtfully deployed. In the case of the community care centre with wet floors, a structured inspection schedule empowered all staff to participate actively rather than leaving hazard detection solely in managerial hands. This inclusive practice fostered ownership and heightened awareness across the team, becoming a vital linchpin in hazard prevention. Similarly, the mental health facility's health surveillance approach, a form of ongoing risk monitoring, enabled the early detection of chemical hazards that manifested subtly across time. These procedures herald the importance of systems that capture both quantitative data and human experiences to present a full hazard landscape.

Incident reporting frameworks are indispensable pillars in hazard identification. The nursing home's swift response to a norovirus outbreak stemmed from an effective system encouraging frontline workers to report even minor or suspected incidents. Such openness dispels the notion that reporting is punitive; rather, it becomes a preventive strategy fostering learning and prompt action. Integral to this process is the culture that nurtures transparent communication and assures staff that their observations and concerns matter. The environmental hazard in the day care centre also benefited from feedback loops, in which families' perspectives identified risks that staff had normalised or unintentionally overlooked. This diversity of input broadens the scope of hazard recognition beyond the professional gaze, reinforcing the principle that hazard identification is a collaborative endeavour embracing all voices within the care network.

Observational skills, both formal and informal, emerged repeatedly as critical facilitators of hazard detection. Whether during routine care, shift handovers, or unstructured moments, frontline staff and managers who cultivate a habit of discerning changes or anomalies contribute immeasurably to safety. The psychological hazards addressed through reflective practice sessions in the residential care unit provide a compelling example: it is in conversation, reflection, and self-awareness that invisible risks surface and invite redress. This practice elevates hazard detection beyond mechanistic checklists into a dynamic interplay of professional insight and human empathy, forming a vital bridge between policy and lived experience.

Ultimately, these case studies advocate for an integrated hazard identification approach, a mosaic where various tools, perspectives, and experiences coalesce to form a comprehensive understanding. The synergy between formal mechanisms, such as inspections and reporting systems, and informal yet equally powerful methods, like observation and feedback, creates a robust safety net. It is within this interplay that health and social care professionals can detect hazards before they precipitate harm and act decisively to mitigate risks.

Moreover, the nuanced reality these examples present is clear: hazards are not static or isolated phenomena but living aspects of complex environments, influenced by human behaviour, organisational culture, physical design, and ever-changing conditions. Recognising this complexity obliges care providers to think creatively and inclusively when examining their contexts, ensuring that no hazard remains unseen due to narrow focus or complacency.

This rich tapestry of real-world experiences deepens understanding and reinforces the idea that effective hazard identification is a skill honed through attentiveness, communication, and a readiness to challenge assumptions. Each case, distinct in its challenges and outcomes, contributes to a broader narrative emphasising that safety in health and social care is an evolving practice one that marries technical proficiency with human connection, vigilance with compassion.

For practitioners, these insights encourage a mindset in which hazard identification is continuous rather than episodic, seamlessly integrated into daily activities and relationships. By embedding tools such as inspections, incident reporting, feedback channels, and reflective observation into the fabric of care, organisations cultivate resilient environments in which hazards are swiftly recognised and addressed. This, in turn, fosters not only safer workplaces but empowers everyone involved to be active participants in safeguarding the dignity, health, and well-being of all who live and work within health and social care settings.

Types of Risks in Health and Social Care

Introduction

Risk is an inherent and unavoidable aspect of health and social care practice. Every day, professionals across the sector make critical decisions that involve balancing safety with the rights, dignity, and independence of individuals receiving care. From my experience working within the sector, I have observed that risk is often misunderstood not simply as something to eliminate, but as something to manage effectively. This distinction is crucial. Overprotective practices can restrict independence, while poor risk management can expose individuals to harm.

Risk assessment, therefore, plays a central role in ensuring safe, effective, and person-centred care. It involves identifying potential hazards, evaluating the likelihood and severity of harm, and implementing control measures to reduce risks to an acceptable level. In the UK, this approach aligns with regulatory frameworks, including those set by the Care Quality Commission (CQC), particularly Regulation 12 (Safe Care and Treatment), which requires providers to assess health and safety risks and take appropriate action to mitigate them.

In practice, risks in health and social care can be broadly categorised into four key areas: environmental, individual, clinical, and organisational. Each category presents unique challenges and requires specific strategies for effective management. Understanding these categories enables practitioners to adopt a structured and proactive approach to risk assessment, ultimately improving outcomes for service users and ensuring compliance with professional standards.

1. Environmental Risks

Environmental risks are hazards present in the physical surroundings where care is delivered. These risks can affect both service users and staff and are often the most visible and immediate concerns in care settings.

1.1 Slips, Trips, and Falls

Slips, trips, and falls are among the most common causes of injury in health and social care environments. They can occur in a variety of settings, including care homes, hospitals, and individuals' homes. Common contributing factors include wet or slippery floors, uneven surfaces, poor lighting, cluttered walkways, and inappropriate footwear.

From my experience in practice, I have noticed that even minor environmental hazards, such as a loose rug or a trailing cable, can lead to serious consequences, particularly for older adults or individuals with mobility challenges. Falls can result in fractures, head injuries, loss of confidence, and, in some cases, long-term disability or death.

Preventive measures include regular environmental checks, prompt cleaning of spills, adequate lighting, use of non-slip flooring, and ensuring walkways are free of obstructions. Risk assessments should also consider individual needs, such as the use of mobility aids or supervision for those at higher risk.

1.2 Unsafe Premises

Unsafe premises pose significant risks to both service users and staff. This includes poorly maintained buildings, faulty equipment, and inadequate safety measures. Examples include broken handrails, damaged flooring, malfunctioning lifts, or inadequate security systems.

I have observed in practice that neglecting routine maintenance can escalate minor issues into major hazards. For instance, a faulty door lock may not only compromise safety but also raise safeguarding concerns, particularly in settings supporting vulnerable individuals.

Ensuring safe premises requires regular inspections, maintenance schedules, and prompt reporting of faults. Organisations must also comply with health and safety legislation, such as the Health and Safety at Work Act 1974, which places a duty on employers to provide a safe working environment.

1.3 Fire Hazards

Fire safety is a critical aspect of environmental risk management. Fire hazards may arise from faulty electrical equipment, improper storage of flammable materials, or failure to adhere to fire safety procedures.

In my experience, fire risk is often underestimated until an incident occurs. However, effective fire safety management can significantly reduce the likelihood and impact of such events. This includes conducting fire risk assessments, maintaining fire detection and alarm systems, ensuring clear evacuation routes, and carrying out regular fire drills.

Staff training is equally important, as all personnel must understand their roles and responsibilities in the event of a fire. This includes knowledge of evacuation procedures, the use of fire extinguishers, and support for individuals with mobility or cognitive impairments during emergencies.

2. Individual Risks

Individual risks are specific to the health conditions, behaviours, and personal circumstances of each service user. These risks require a person-centred approach, as no two individuals present the same level or type of risk.

2.1 Falls Risk

Falls risk is particularly prevalent among older adults and individuals with physical or cognitive impairments. Factors contributing to falls include muscle weakness, balance issues, medication side effects, visual impairment, and environmental hazards.

From my observations, falls are rarely caused by a single factor; rather, they result from a combination of intrinsic and extrinsic elements. For example, an individual taking sedative medication may become dizzy, increasing their likelihood of falling, especially in a poorly lit environment.

Effective management involves comprehensive risk assessments, the use of mobility aids, regular monitoring, and tailored care plans. Encouraging safe mobility rather than restricting movement is essential to maintaining independence and dignity.

2.2 Self-Harm

Self-harm is a significant risk among individuals with mental health conditions. It may manifest in various forms, including physical injury or neglect of personal well-being.

In my practice, I have noticed that managing self-harm risk requires a sensitive and holistic approach. It is not sufficient to simply remove hazards; practitioners must also address underlying emotional and psychological factors.

Risk management strategies include regular observation, development of personalised care plans, involvement of mental health professionals, and effective communication with the individual. Safeguarding procedures must also be followed where there is a risk of serious harm.

2.3 Malnutrition

Malnutrition is a common yet often overlooked risk in health and social care settings. It can result from poor appetite, medical conditions, swallowing difficulties, or lack of support with eating and drinking.

I have observed that malnutrition can develop gradually and may not be immediately apparent. However, its consequences can be severe, including weight loss, weakened immune function, delayed recovery, and increased risk of infection.

Assessment tools such as the Malnutrition Universal Screening Tool (MUST) are commonly used to identify individuals at risk. Interventions may include dietary support, monitoring food and fluid intake, and involving dietitians where necessary.

3. Clinical Risks

Clinical risks arise from healthcare interventions, treatments, and procedures. These risks require a high level of competence, adherence to protocols, and continuous monitoring.

3.1 Medication Errors

Medication errors are a significant concern in health and social care. These errors can occur at any stage, including prescribing, dispensing, and administration.

From my experience, common causes of medication errors include poor communication, lack of training, workload pressures, and inadequate documentation. The consequences can range from minor side effects to serious harm or death.

To reduce this risk, practitioners must adhere to established protocols, including the "five rights" of medication administration. Regular training, supervision, and audits are also essential.

3.2 Infection Control Issues

Infection prevention and control are fundamental aspects of safe care. Poor practices can lead to the spread of infections, particularly in vulnerable populations.

I have noticed that simple measures such as hand hygiene, use of personal protective equipment (PPE), and proper cleaning procedures can significantly reduce infection risks. However, these measures must be consistently applied.

Organisations must have clear policies in place, and staff must receive regular training to ensure compliance with best practices.

3.3 Moving and Handling Injuries

Moving and handling activities present risks to both staff and service users. Incorrect techniques can result in musculoskeletal injuries for staff and physical harm to individuals.

In practice, I have observed that injuries often occur when staff attempt to move individuals without proper equipment or training. This highlights the importance of risk assessments, the use of appropriate equipment, and adherence to safe techniques.

4. Organisational Risks

Organisational risks relate to the systems, structures, and processes within a care service. These risks can have a significant impact on the quality and safety of care delivery.

4.1 Staff Shortages

Staff shortages are a major challenge in the health and social care sector. Insufficient staffing levels can lead to increased workload, stress, and reduced quality of care.

From my experience, staff shortages often result in missed care tasks, delayed responses, and increased risk of errors. This can compromise the safety and well-being of service users.

Effective workforce planning, recruitment strategies, and staff retention initiatives are essential to address this issue.

4.2 Poor Communication

Communication is a critical component of safe care. Poor communication can lead to misunderstandings, errors, and adverse outcomes.

I have noticed that many incidents in practice can be traced back to communication failures, particularly during handovers or when documentation is incomplete.

Improving communication requires clear protocols, effective training, and a culture that encourages openness and accountability.

4.3 Lack of Training

A lack of training can significantly increase the risk of poor practice. Staff who are not adequately trained may lack the knowledge and skills required to perform their roles safely and effectively.

In my role as an assessor, I have seen how continuous professional development can enhance competence and confidence among staff. Training should cover key areas such as safeguarding, medication management, infection control, and risk assessment.

Conclusion

In conclusion, understanding the different types of risks in health and social care is essential for delivering safe, effective, and person-centred services. Environmental, individual, clinical, and organisational risks each present unique challenges that require careful assessment and management.

From my experience, effective risk management is not about eliminating risk entirely but about making informed decisions that balance safety with independence. This requires a proactive approach, strong leadership, and a commitment to continuous improvement.

By recognising and addressing these risks, health and social care professionals can create safer environments, enhance the quality of care, and ultimately make a meaningful difference in the lives of those they support.

Risk Assessment Process

The 5 Steps to Risk Assessment

Embarking on the journey of risk assessment is, at its core, an exercise in foresight and prudence, a meticulous process designed to safeguard those within health and social care environments while fostering an atmosphere in which care flourishes without the undue burden of fear or restriction. The five essential steps to risk assessment form a structured pathway, each phase building upon the previous, culminating in a robust, dynamic understanding of the risks present and the strategies necessary to manage them effectively. It is through this process that care providers can transform abstract concepts of safety into tangible, actionable measures that protect service users, staff, and ultimately the integrity of the care setting itself.

The first and foundational step is the identification of hazards, an exercise that demands not only vigilance but also a comprehensive appreciation of the many dimensions in which harm can arise. Hazards, in this context, refer to any element, condition, or practice within the workplace that has the potential to cause injury, ill-health, or damage. This identification process transcends the obvious physical dangers often visualised, such as slippery floors or faulty equipment, to embrace a wider spectrum, including biological hazards, such as infectious agents; chemical risks from exposure to harmful substances; environmental challenges, such as extreme temperatures; and psychological factors, such as stress and workplace bullying. The challenge lies in cultivating a mindset that anticipates the less visible or immediate dangers, understanding that risks in health and social care are as varied as the human conditions under care. This step requires active engagement with the environment through detailed workplace inspections, consultations with staff and service users, and feedback mechanisms. By incorporating the insights of those who operate daily within the care setting, a richer, more nuanced picture of hazards emerges, one that respects the experiential knowledge of front-line workers and service users alike.

Once hazards are identified, the process naturally flows to determine who might be harmed and how. This second step is pivotal; risk assessment is not merely about cataloguing dangers but understanding their potential impact on individuals. Here, the emphasis is on exploring the spectrum of people at risk, not only the service users who may be vulnerable due to illness or disability, but also care providers, visitors, support staff, and even contractors. Each group experiences risk differently, shaped by underlying health, capability, and proximity to hazards. A frail elderly person, for instance, may be particularly susceptible to falls, while a care worker might face ergonomic injuries during manual handling tasks. Similarly, some hazards may disproportionately affect individuals with sensory impairments or cognitive conditions. Beyond identifying who is at risk, this phase delves deeper into the nature of potential harm, whether it be physical injury, mental distress, or exposure to infectious diseases. Such understanding enables tailored risk management strategies that acknowledge and respect the individuality of those involved, steering clear of one-size-fits-all solutions and promoting dignity and empowerment.

Armed with knowledge of hazards and their potential victims, the third step calls for evaluating the risks essentially, scrutinising the likelihood and severity of harm to prioritise where efforts and resources should be concentrated. Evaluation is as much an art as a science, requiring the integration of evidence, professional judgement, and contextual awareness. At this juncture, a risk matrix becomes an invaluable tool, translating complex variables into a visual framework that guides decision-making. The common approach within health and social care settings involves assessing risk by pairing the probability of an adverse event occurring against the magnitude of its consequences. For example, a rare event that could cause catastrophic injury would be ranked as high risk and warrant immediate attention, while a frequent event causing minor inconvenience might be categorised as low risk. This binary analysis fosters clarity and helps avoid paralysis by detail, enabling care teams to allocate resources toward interventions that will yield the greatest impact in safeguarding individuals. However, the evaluation process must also account for the dynamic nature of health and social care environments, where risks evolve with changing service user needs, new treatments, or shifting operational conditions, underscoring the importance of flexibility and ongoing reassessment.

The fourth step, recording the findings, may seem a procedural formality, yet it holds profound significance in creating an accountable and transparent culture. Documenting risk assessments furnishes a tangible record that communicates to all stakeholders the hazards recognised, who is at risk, the evaluation outcomes, and the control measures implemented. This documentation is a living artefact; it provides a baseline for training, informs emergency responses, supports compliance with legal requirements, and promotes a shared understanding of safety priorities. Effective recording transcends mere note-taking; it should be clear, concise, and accessible, avoiding jargon where possible, and tailored to the specific needs of the care environment. It should also capture the rationale behind judgments made and actions taken, offering insight into the thought processes that underpin risk management decisions. Involving service users and staff in this documentation process, where appropriate, can reinforce ownership and encourage a proactive safety culture. Moreover, meticulous records become invaluable during inspections by regulatory agents, serving as evidence of due diligence and continuous commitment to quality care.

Finally, the fifth step, the review of risk assessments, is the crucible in which the process's enduring value is forged. Risk assessments are not static snapshots; rather, they must be living documents, regularly revisited and updated to reflect changes in care practices, environments, or service user conditions. The review process embodies the principle of continuous improvement, inviting reflection on the effectiveness of current controls and opening the door to innovation or adaptation. Scheduled revisits should align with organisational policies but also be responsive to incidents, near misses, audits, and feedback from all levels of the care workforce. A comprehensive review scrutinises whether hazards have altered, whether the demographics or vulnerabilities of service users have shifted, and whether new hazards have emerged, such as those arising from novel treatments or technologies. Additionally, it reevaluates the assigned risk ratings, acknowledging that both likelihood and severity can fluctuate over time. This iterative cycle cultivates resilience within the organisation, ensuring risk management practices remain relevant and robust, underpinning the safety and dignity of care delivery.

Throughout this five-step journey, the integration of practical tools such as risk matrices underpins a systematic approach to prioritising hazards, transforming the sometimes nebulous concept of risk into actionable intelligence. By visually mapping the interplay between likelihood and impact, care providers are equipped to navigate complex decision-making landscapes with confidence and clarity. This methodological discipline does not diminish the compassionate aspect of care but rather enhances it, providing a framework that supports proactive measures and enables measured positive risk-taking, encouraging independence while maintaining vigilance. The meticulous identification of hazards, thoughtful consideration of those at risk, precise evaluation of potential harm, thorough documentation, and committed review collectively construct a resilient sheath of protection around all stakeholders in health and social care. Embracing these five steps with rigour and empathy ultimately empowers care professionals not only to manage risks but to transform them into opportunities for improved safety, dignity, and quality of life.

Risk Rating and Scoring

Risk rating and scoring are the pivotal stage where raw data from hazard identification and risk analysis transform into actionable insights that steer decision-making in health and social care environments. This process involves a nuanced evaluation of each identified risk's likelihood of occurrence and the severity of its potential consequences. Balancing these two dimensions allows care professionals to not only comprehend the magnitude of each risk but also prioritise their efforts efficiently, ensuring that limited resources are allocated where they can make the most significant difference to safety and well-being. At its heart, risk rating is a sophisticated yet practical exercise in judgment, combining quantitative measures and qualitative understanding to unravel the complex tapestry of everyday risks faced within health and social care settings.

Understanding likelihood involves assessing how probable it is that a particular hazard will cause harm. This is not a straightforward calculation but rather an expression of probability based on experience, current environmental factors, and the specific context in which care is delivered. For example, the likelihood of a patient falling in a busy care home depends on factors such as mobility impairments, environmental hazards like slippery floors, and the presence or absence of supervision. Likelihood is not static; it can fluctuate in response to changes in conditions, staff attentiveness, or the implementation of control measures. Often, likelihood is categorised into gradations such as 'rare,' 'unlikely,' 'possible,' 'likely,' and 'almost certain,' each describing an increasingly frequent chance of occurrence. Determining where a risk falls on this scale requires practitioners to draw on observation, data recording, and sometimes intuition cultivated through experience. It's essential to recognise that overestimating or underestimating likelihood can have serious repercussions; overestimating might lead to unnecessary restrictions or resource deployment, while underestimating can leave hazards unchecked and persons at risk.

Severity, the other cornerstone of risk rating, examines the potential impact or harm that could arise if the risk materialises. In health and social care, severity is entwined with both physical harm and psychological, emotional, or social consequences experienced by service users and staff alike. It extends beyond the immediate effects to consider longer-term outcomes such as prolonged recovery, loss of independence, or emotional trauma. Severity scales often range from 'insignificant' or 'minor' harm, such as a small bruise or discomfort, to 'catastrophic,' which might entail permanent disability, death, or significant legal liabilities. Unlike likelihood, severity is less prone to frequent changes once a hazard is identified, as it fundamentally reflects the nature of the potential harm. Nonetheless, it too demands careful contemplation, particularly in balancing the tangible and intangible effects on individuals' dignity and quality of life. For example, a medication error may seem quantitatively minor but could have catastrophic consequences depending on the medication involved.

The intersection of likelihood and severity forms the foundation for risk matrices, a universally embraced tool that facilitates the prioritisation of risks in systematic and transparent ways. A risk matrix typically presents a grid, with likelihood on one axis and severity on the other, subdivided into cells representing different levels of risk. This visual framework enables straightforward plotting of each identified risk based on its assigned likelihood and severity ratings, which in turn yields a composite risk score or category. The cells are usually colour-coded, ranging from green for low-risk scenarios where the combination poses negligible threats, through amber for medium risk necessitating monitoring and mitigatory action, to red signifying high risks where urgent intervention is required. By reducing complex assessments to visual, easy-to-recognise formats, risk matrices empower care providers and managers to make quick relative-risk comparisons and communicate priorities across diverse teams.

However, the use of risk matrices is not just about ticking boxes but involves a deeper analytical engagement. It necessitates rigorous and consistent application of definitions for likelihood and severity to assure reliability and fairness across assessments. For instance, what qualifies as 'likely' in one care setting may not equate to 'likely' in another, depending on organisational culture, available resources, and experience. Similarly, subjective biases or emotional responses to risks must be managed carefully to maintain objectivity. Effective training and clear guidelines are indispensable to underpin uniform application, ensuring that risk matrices serve genuine prioritisation rather than a mechanical exercise. Moreover, risk matrices can accommodate additional complexity; some models incorporate weighting factors or thresholds to address sensitivities, such as risks involving vulnerable populations or high-profile service users.

Once risks are plotted and scored, prioritisation becomes an actionable strategy. This requires an understanding that not all risks demand equal attention. Risks rated with high likelihood and severe consequences naturally command immediate and comprehensive controls. Conversely, those with low likelihood and low severity might be deemed acceptable or monitored with minimal intervention, freeing resources for more pressing hazards. However, the process must retain flexibility to reflect evolving conditions and remain open to reassessment. For instance, a low-likelihood risk might escalate rapidly if a new medication regimen is introduced or a patient's health deteriorates, necessitating an agile response. The prioritisation framework fosters a dynamic risk management approach, guiding the deployment of training, equipment, supervision, and policy changes based on quantified risk profiles.

Beyond immediate risk ranking, risk rating, and scoring underpin deeper strategic objectives. They feed into organisational reporting, compliance documentation, and benchmarking efforts, providing verifiable evidence of the systematic approach to safeguarding. Risk registers and risk assessment reports, constructed from these scores, serve as critical communication tools, facilitating dialogue among management, care teams, regulators, and even service users and their families. Transparent risk scoring supports shared understanding, collective ownership, and collaborative problem-solving, vital for sustaining positive risk cultures. Moreover, it empowers meaningful involvement of service users by enabling clearer explanations of risk levels and justifications for care decisions, thereby reinforcing respect and dignity.

Despite their strengths, critics sometimes caution against overreliance on risk matrices and scoring, warning that they can obscure the subtleties of individual circumstances and reduce complex human realities to simplistic figures. While scoring offers valuable guidance, it must be integrated with professional judgment, ethical reflection, and person-centred assessments that consider service users' holistic well-being. For example, a risk with moderate numerical scores might still require urgent action if it threatens a service user's autonomy or if the person perceives an unacceptable threat to their safety. Harmonising quantitative risk-rating tools with these qualitative insights is at the heart of effective risk management in health and social care.

Ultimately, the skilful application of likelihood-versus-severity assessments, coupled with the adept use of risk matrices, equips care providers with a clear, systematic pathway to identify which hazards demand urgent correction and which can be managed with routine vigilance. This clarity fosters confidence in navigating risk, alleviates anxiety among staff, and cultivates a culture where positive risk-taking is balanced against safety imperatives. As care environments grow increasingly complex, with diverse service user needs and regulatory demands, mastering risk rating and scoring becomes not just a technical requirement but a vital element in delivering compassionate, high-quality care that protects and empowers all involved.

Applying Risk Assessment Models

In practical health and social care settings, applying risk assessment models transforms theoretical frameworks into real-world tools that safeguard service users while supporting care providers' professional judgment. The process is far from a mere checklist exercise; it demands a nuanced understanding of the environment, the people involved, and the unpredictable nature of human health and behaviour. This dynamic interplay challenges care professionals to use risk assessment models not simply as bureaucratic requirements but as living instruments guiding daily decisions. To bring this to life, we will explore how these models operate step by step, weaving in examples that illuminate their practical applications and the decision-making that underpins effective risk management.

At the heart of most models is the classic five-step framework: identifying hazards, assessing the risks associated with those hazards, deciding on control measures, implementing those controls, and finally, reviewing and revisiting the assessment to ensure it remains valid. In health and social care, these steps must be applied with acute sensitivity to the individual needs and rights of service users, as risks extend beyond physical to emotional, psychological, and social.

Consider the task of assessing fall risk in a residential care home. The first step, identifying hazards, requires a comprehensive survey of the environment in tandem with an evaluation of service users' mobility, cognitive state, and any medications that might affect balance or alertness. Here, the hazard is not simply the presence of slippery floors or uneven surfaces, but also the vulnerability of the individual resident as they move through that space. A care worker might observe that a particular resident uses a walking frame intermittently and has occasional episodes of dizziness. This identification extends beyond physical hazards to the complex interplay between personal vulnerability and environmental factors.

Once hazards are identified, the next step is to assess the risk by evaluating the likelihood and severity of harm occurring. This is where risk matrices come into play. These tools allow practitioners to systematically rank risks, clarifying which require immediate attention and which can be monitored. Using the falls example, a likelihood-versus-severity matrix helps quantify whether a resident with moderate balance issues who slips once is a medium or low risk, depending on past incident history and environmental safeguards. The matrix might indicate a high likelihood of a fall occurring, and because the potential harm could be severe, such as fractures or head injuries, the overall risk rating escalates, signalling the need for swift action.

With risk levels established, deciding on control measures becomes paramount. In our scenario, this could involve multiple layers of interventions: installing non-slip mats, introducing a scheduled supervision system during high-risk activities like bathing or moving between rooms, or consulting with physiotherapists to develop strength and balance exercises. Importantly, the control measures must be reasonable and proportionate, consistently balancing safety with the resident's independence and dignity. Applying a control that overly restricts mobility to prevent falls might cause harm through loss of confidence, muscle atrophy, or social isolation. Therefore, thoughtful deliberation guides which interventions not only mitigate risk but also promote well-being and autonomy.

Implementation is where theoretical strategies meet practical realities. The success of controls depends on effective communication among staff, appropriate training, and the organisation's commitment to fostering a positive risk culture. Documentation plays a critical role here, recording exactly what control measures have been adopted, who is responsible for monitoring them, and setting clear timelines for re-assessment. Imagine a care manager overseeing this: they organise team briefings to ensure everyone understands the new supervision routines and environmental adjustments, and encourage staff to report any emerging issues or near-misses promptly. This culture of vigilance and openness supports continuous learning and adaptation.

Reviewing the risk assessment closes the loop and highlights that risk management is an evolving process. As residents' conditions change, perhaps a resident's mobility improves with therapy or declines due to illness, the risk level fluctuates, necessitating updated control measures. Reviews might be triggered by events such as falls or changes in medication or be scheduled regularly as part of governance practices. This cyclical approach underscores that risk assessment is not static but must respond dynamically to the realities of care environments.

Beyond the classic five-step process, care professionals often benefit from applying more nuanced or specialised models tailored to their unique contexts. One such example is the use of the Bowtie Model, which graphically represents risk by linking potential causes to consequences with barriers (controls) designed to prevent or mitigate harm. In a mental health inpatient setting, this model can clarify complex risks such as self-harm or aggression. Causes may include triggers like medication side effects, environmental stressors, or social isolation. Barriers might be trained staff intervention, environmental design modifications to reduce isolation, or therapy programs. Visualising this interplay ensures that care workers understand not only what risks exist but also how various measures interconnect to prevent incidents.

Moreover, the use of Failure Modes and Effects Analysis (FMEA) introduces a proactive, systematic approach to risk by identifying how processes might fail and assessing the impact of these failure points. For example, in medication administration, FMEA encourages a review of every step from prescription to delivery, anticipating errors like incorrect dosage or timing. Care teams assign scores based on the severity of potential harm, the frequency of occurrence, and the likelihood of detection before harm ensues. Such detailed analysis aids in targeting process weaknesses and tailoring controls, such as double-check systems or electronic alarms for missed doses.

Another important consideration when applying risk assessment models is the role of documentation as both a safeguard and a communication tool. Practical examples demonstrate that poorly documented risk assessments, no matter how thorough, lose impact and may even result in regulatory censure. A care provider visiting a service user's home must write clear, accessible notes outlining the identified hazards, risk ratings, control actions, and the rationale for decisions, ensuring transparency for colleagues and external agencies such as the Care Quality Commission. This documentation also supports continuity of care, allowing new or temporary staff to pick up the risk management strategy without delay or confusion.

In community care, the dynamic nature of settings demands the frequent use of dynamic risk assessments and real-time evaluations conducted in fluid or unpredictable scenarios. A domiciliary care worker might enter a service user's home and immediately spot a new hazard, such as a wet floor, increased clutter, or indications of distress in the service user. Applying risk assessment models in such moments entails rapid hazard identification and risk rating, followed by instant decision-making, perhaps postponing physically demanding tasks or requesting assistance. This agility exemplifies the practical value of these frameworks beyond static paper documents, embedding risk awareness into everyday practice.

Case studies illustrate how risk assessment models also facilitate negotiation of positive risk-taking. For instance, an elderly service user with mild cognitive impairment might wish to prepare their meals independently despite some risk of minor burns or cuts. The model supports a structured discussion where hazards are identified and weighted against the benefits of autonomy, well-being, and quality of life. Strategies might include installing accessible safety devices, training the individual carefully, and arranging periodic monitoring visits. Here, the risk assessment model serves as a tool for empowerment, enabling professionals to support individuality and dignity while managing safety concerns.

Instances of multi-agency collaboration are further enriched when risk assessments are standardised through common models. When social workers, nursing staff, occupational therapists, and family members share a clear, visual risk framework, such as a unified risk matrix, communication improves significantly. This alignment fosters consistent understanding and coordinated action plans, avoiding fragmented approaches that compromise safety. For example, in safeguarding vulnerable adults, a risk matrix highlighting escalating concerns allows all parties to prioritise interventions coherently, share responsibilities, and reduce the likelihood of oversight.

Training care staff in the application of risk assessment models is essential for successful implementation. Practical workshops that walk through realistic scenarios enable practitioners to internalise the steps of hazard identification, risk rating, and control selection. Role-playing exercises help embed confidence in making subjective judgments about likelihood and impact, grounded in evidence and best practice. Over time, these skills develop into an intuitive part of professional judgment, combining the art and science of safer care.

An additional practical dimension of applying risk assessment models lies in integrating technological tools that support and document the process. Digital platforms can host risk assessments, triggering alerts for review dates, escalating risks, or deviations from control implementation. For example, tablet-based apps allow care workers to input observational data in real time, cross-reference risk matrices, and access guidance prompts on control measures. This technology not only streamlines the process but also enhances accuracy, reduces paperwork, and fosters accountability.

Ethical considerations permeate the application of risk assessment models. Care providers must navigate tensions between minimising risk and respecting the service user's rights to autonomy and freedom. Models that focus exclusively on eliminating risk may inadvertently lead to overprotection and deprivation of choice. Therefore, applying these frameworks requires a holistic perspective that incorporates the principles of person-centred care, informed consent, and shared decision-making. The risk assessment process becomes a dialogue rather than a unilateral judgment, balancing evidence-based safety with respect for individual values.

In conclusion, the application of risk assessment models in health and social care is a sophisticated practice that demands flexibility, insight, and collaboration. Practical examples reveal the multifaceted nature of hazards, the necessity for precise risk evaluation through matrices and analytical tools, and the thoughtful deployment of control measures that do not compromise dignity. Dynamic assessments, multi-agency communication, and technological integration synergise to make risk management an active and responsive endeavour. Above all, risk assessment models empower professionals to embrace positive risk-taking, fostering environments where safety coexists with independence, respect, and human flourishing. This ongoing journey from theoretical framework to lived practice is what makes risk assessment not just a process, but a transformative element of quality care.

Risk Matrix and Control Measures in Health and Social Care

Risk assessment is a fundamental component of safe and effective practice in health and social care. From my experience working within the sector, I have noticed that risk is present in almost every aspect of care delivery, whether it relates to the environment, the individual, clinical interventions, or organisational systems. The challenge for practitioners is not to eliminate risk, as this is neither realistic nor desirable, but to manage it effectively to promote safety while preserving dignity and independence.

A structured approach to risk assessment is essential in achieving this balance. One of the most widely used tools in practice is the risk assessment matrix, which enables practitioners to evaluate risks based on their likelihood and severity. This process supports informed decision-making and helps prioritise actions to minimise harm.

Alongside risk assessment, the implementation of appropriate control measures is equally important. These measures are designed to reduce or eliminate risks and ensure that care is delivered in a safe and controlled manner. In my role, I have found that the effectiveness of risk management depends not only on identifying risks but also on applying the right control strategies and reviewing them regularly.

This chapter explores the key components of the risk assessment matrix, including likelihood, severity, and risk levels, as well as the hierarchy of control measures used to manage risks in health and social care settings.

Understanding the Risk Assessment Matrix

A risk assessment matrix is a practical tool for evaluating the level of risk associated with a particular hazard. It combines two key factors: the likelihood of an event occurring and the severity of its potential consequences. By analysing these elements, practitioners can determine the overall level of risk and decide on appropriate actions.

In my experience, using a risk matrix brings structure and consistency to the assessment process. It helps practitioners to move beyond subjective judgment and adopt a more systematic approach. It also supports communication within teams, as risks can be clearly categorised and prioritised.

The matrix typically categorises risks into three main levels: low, medium, and high. These levels guide decision-making and ensure that resources are allocated effectively.

Likelihood of Risk

Likelihood refers to the probability that a particular risk will occur. In practice, likelihood is influenced by various factors, including the environment, the individual's condition, and the effectiveness of existing control measures.

Low Likelihood

A low likelihood indicates that the risk is unlikely to occur. This may be due to effective control measures already in place or because the hazard is rarely encountered.

From what I have observed, low-likelihood risks are often present in well-managed environments where procedures are consistently followed. For example, the risk of slips in a well-maintained care home with non-slip flooring and regular cleaning may be considered low.

However, it is important not to ignore low-likelihood risks. Even unlikely events can occur, and when they do, they may still have significant consequences.

Medium Likelihood

A medium likelihood suggests that the risk could occur under certain circumstances. This is often the case where control measures exist but may not always be effective or consistently applied.

In my experience, many risks in health and social care fall into this category. For example, medication errors may be considered a medium likelihood due to factors such as workload, communication issues, or human error.

Managing medium-likelihood risks requires ongoing monitoring and reinforcement of control measures.

High Likelihood

A high likelihood indicates that the risk is very likely to occur or has occurred frequently in the past. These risks require immediate attention and robust control measures.

I have noticed that high-likelihood risks often arise in situations where there are systemic issues, such as staff shortages or a lack of training. For example, frequent incidents of falls in a care setting may indicate a high risk that needs urgent intervention.

Severity of Risk

Severity refers to the potential impact or consequences of a risk if it occurs. It is essential to consider not only the likelihood of an event but also how serious the outcome could be.

Minor Severity

Minor severity involves low-level harm or minimal impact. This may include minor injuries, temporary discomfort, or slight inconvenience.

From my experience, minor risks are common in everyday care activities. For example, a small bruise from a minor fall may be considered a minor outcome.

While these risks may not require extensive intervention, they should still be monitored to prevent escalation.

Moderate Severity

Moderate severity involves more significant harm that may require medical attention or result in temporary impairment.

Examples include fractures, infections, or moderate emotional distress. In practice, these risks can have a noticeable impact on an individual's well-being and may require additional support.

I have observed that moderate risks often highlight gaps in existing control measures and should prompt a review of practices.

Severe Severity

Severe severity involves serious harm, long-term disability, or even death. These risks are of greatest concern and require immediate, comprehensive management.

Examples include life-threatening injuries, serious safeguarding incidents, or major clinical errors.

From my perspective, severe risks must always be prioritised, regardless of their likelihood, because of their potential consequences.

Risk Levels

By combining likelihood and severity, practitioners can determine the overall risk level. This helps prioritise actions and allocate resources effectively.

Low Risk

Low-risk situations involve minimal likelihood and/or minor severity. These risks can generally be managed through routine procedures and monitoring.

In my experience, low risks should not be ignored but managed proportionately. Overreacting to low risks can lead to unnecessary restrictions.

Medium Risk

Medium risks require more attention and may need additional control measures. These risks should be monitored regularly and reviewed to ensure they do not escalate.

I have found that effective communication and teamwork are essential in managing medium risks.

High Risk

High risks involve either a high likelihood or severe consequences, or both. These risks require immediate action and robust control measures.

From my experience, failure to address high risks promptly can lead to serious incidents and regulatory concerns.

Control Strategies in Risk Management

Once risks have been identified and assessed, appropriate control measures must be implemented. The hierarchy of control provides a structured approach to managing risks, prioritising the most effective methods.

Elimination

Elimination involves removing the hazard entirely. This is the most effective control measure as it eliminates the risk at its source.

For example, removing faulty equipment from use eliminates the risk of injury.

In my experience, elimination is not always possible, particularly in care settings where certain risks are inherent. However, where it is feasible, it should always be the first option considered.

Substitution

Substitution involves replacing a hazard with a safer alternative. This reduces risk while still allowing activities to continue.

For example, using safer cleaning products instead of hazardous chemicals.

I have noticed that substitution is particularly useful in reducing environmental and clinical risks.

Engineering Controls

Engineering controls involve the use of equipment or physical changes to reduce risk. This includes tools, devices, or environmental modifications.

Examples include hoists for moving and handling, bed rails, and alarm systems.

From my experience, engineering controls are highly effective as they do not rely solely on human behaviour.

Administrative Controls

Administrative controls involve policies, procedures, training, and supervision. These measures guide behaviour and ensure that risks are managed consistently.

Examples include risk assessments, staff training, and standard operating procedures.

I have found that administrative controls are essential but must be supported by a strong organisational culture to be effective.

Personal Protective Equipment (PPE)

PPE includes items such as gloves, masks, and aprons that protect individuals from harm.

While PPE is important, it is considered the least effective control measure as it relies on correct use by individuals.

In my experience, PPE should always be used alongside other control measures rather than as a standalone solution.

Applying the Risk Matrix in Practice

In practice, the risk matrix is used as part of a broader risk assessment process. This involves identifying hazards, evaluating risks, implementing controls, and reviewing outcomes.

I have observed that effective use of the risk matrix requires training, consistency, and regular review. It should not be a one-off exercise but an ongoing process.

Challenges in Risk Assessment

There are several challenges associated with risk assessment, including subjectivity, lack of training, and organisational pressures.

From my experience, one of the biggest challenges is achieving consistency across different practitioners.

Conclusion

In conclusion, the risk matrix and control measures are essential tools in managing risk in health and social care. They provide a structured approach to identifying, assessing, and mitigating risks.

From my perspective, effective risk management requires a combination of knowledge, judgement, and continuous improvement.

By applying these principles, practitioners can create safer environments, improve outcomes, and make a meaningful difference in the lives of those they support.

Managing and Controlling Risks

Control Measures

In the multifaceted realm of health and social care, implementing effective control measures stands as the cornerstone of safeguarding both service users and care providers. Risk, by its very nature, is an inherent element of human environments, yet the art and science of risk management lie in judiciously applying a spectrum of interventions designed to minimise potential harm without unduly restricting the dignity and autonomy of those in care. Control measures are, therefore, not merely procedural steps; they embody a dynamic, evolving approach that balances precaution with practicality, rooted in a disciplined understanding of risk hierarchy and responsive adaptability.

At the apex of control strategies lies elimination, the most robust and sought-after measure in any risk management plan. Elimination involves completely removing the hazard from the environment or process, thereby obliterating the risk it poses. Within health and social care settings, this might translate into redesigning tasks to exclude hazardous steps, removing harmful substances, or transitioning away from outdated equipment known to cause accidents. Although theoretically straightforward, elimination often demands significant resources, systemic change, or cultural shifts within an organisation. Its success hinges on thorough hazard identification and a commitment from all levels of the care workforce to embrace transformative change. Eliminating the need for manual lifting by introducing hoists, removing toxic chemicals by substituting less harmful alternatives, or streamlining processes to reduce exposure to infection are prime examples of this intervention's power to fundamentally alter outcomes.

When elimination is not feasible, substitution emerges as the next stratagem in the risk control hierarchy. This measure involves replacing hazardous materials, equipment, or procedures with less dangerous alternatives. Substitution requires a nuanced understanding of risk; the replacement must genuinely diminish harm without introducing new, unforeseen hazards. For instance, substituting a cleaning agent that contains harsh chemicals with a biodegradable, less toxic formula can reduce both the environmental impact and worker exposure to irritants. Similarly, substituting bulky, complicated machinery with user-friendly, safer technology can reduce the likelihood of operator error and injury. However, substitution demands continuous vigilance, as replacements must be frequently reassessed for efficacy and unforeseen consequences. It is not a one-time fix but an ongoing commitment to improvement, intertwined with training, education, and feedback mechanisms.

Engineering controls represent a different layer of defence, predicated on physically isolating people from hazards or modifying the work environment to mitigate risk. In health and social care, this can mean installing handrails, implementing safer architectural designs, or incorporating mechanical aids to reduce manual handling. Engineering controls also encompass ventilation systems designed to reduce airborne contaminants or secure storage facilities that minimise the risk of unintended exposure to medicines or chemicals. The elegance of engineering controls lies in their ability to create systemic, passive protections, reducing reliance on human behaviour and decisions of care, which are often subject to variability and human error. These interventions demand substantial investment in planning, infrastructure, and maintenance but deliver continuous, proactive safety benefits.

Administrative controls form the organisational scaffold that supports all other risk control measures. They operate through policies, procedures, training, supervision, and work scheduling that influence how tasks are performed and how hazards are recognised and responded to. Administrative controls ensure that the organisational culture promotes safety as a shared responsibility and embeds risk assessment in daily practice. These measures are highly adaptable and vital in settings where hazards are dynamic or where elimination, substitution, or engineering controls are insufficient or impractical. Developing comprehensive policies that clearly outline safe operating procedures, ensuring staff receive thorough induction and role-tailored refresher training, and scheduling regular risk assessments and audits all fall within this administrative domain. Moreover, promoting open communication channels for reporting concerns or near misses fosters a preventative, learning-oriented environment. Cultural factors heavily influence the effectiveness of administrative controls; they require leadership commitment, transparency, and empowering all team members to cultivate a climate in which safety is actively pursued, and failures become opportunities for improvement rather than sources of blame.

Personal Protective Equipment (PPE) represents the final barrier of defence, intended to protect individuals when hazards cannot be adequately controlled by other means or as supplementary protection. PPE includes items such as gloves, masks, gowns, eye protection, and specialised footwear, all designed to prevent direct exposure to infectious agents, hazardous substances, or physical injury. In health and social care, the use of PPE is of profound significance, especially in the context of infection control, biochemical hazards, or aggressive behaviour. However, the effectiveness of PPE is heavily contingent upon correct selection, fitting, use, maintenance, and disposal. It is therefore essential to embed comprehensive training and compliance monitoring into PPE programs. Despite its prominence, PPE should never be regarded as a primary or sole control measure, as its protective capacity depends on individual adherence and can fail if improperly managed. Its role is critical, but it must be framed within a multi-layered risk-control strategy that prioritises systemic interventions.

Safe systems of work are the dynamic conjunction of administrative, engineering, substitution, and elimination controls, underpinned by organisational commitment and continual workforce engagement. They emerge from a systematic approach in which tasks are analysed for risks, controls are selected based on the hierarchy of risk-control principles, and procedures are embedded through training, supervision, and policy enforcement. A safe system proactively anticipates hazards and plans for contingencies, rather than merely reacting to incidents. It includes emergency response plans, clear communication protocols, and incident reporting mechanisms, ensuring that risk management adapts responsively to new challenges, emerging threats, and lessons learned from past events. Moreover, these systems recognise the human element in risk, offering support, education, and involvement to those who execute and are affected by risk assessments and controls. When workers feel empowered and informed, compliance increases, as does the capacity for innovation in safety practices.

Dynamic risk assessment complements safe systems of work by offering a flexible, real-time evaluation of risk in rapidly changing or unpredictable environments typical of health and social care settings where emergencies and complex situations abound. Unlike formal risk assessments, which are planned and documented, dynamic risk assessment is an ongoing mental process that care providers use as they navigate day-to-day care tasks. It requires astute observation, quick judgment, and the ability to modify actions proactively in response to evolving conditions. For instance, when assisting a service user who suddenly becomes unsteady, a care provider must reassess potential risks and adapt their support, calling for increased vigilance, adjusting positioning, or summoning help. In critical incidents such as outbreaks of infectious disease, sudden staff shortages, or environmental hazards like fire or flood, dynamic risk assessments are indispensable for mitigating harm. Training staff to develop these skills, encouraging a mindset of constant awareness, and embedding protocols that support rapid decision-making are central to enhancing this capability.

Collectively, these control measures form an interwoven framework that underpins excellence and safety in health and social care risk management. The true strength lies not in any one measure alone but in their synergistic application, undergirded by continuous evaluation and a culture that values safety, dignity, and empowerment equally. Through the elimination of hazards, substitution with safer alternatives, implementation of engineering solutions, robust administrative controls, and judicious use of personal protective equipment, care providers gain the tools and confidence to navigate complex environments where risk is a constant companion. Coupled with dynamic risk assessment and a commitment to maintaining safe systems of work, these measures enable health and social care professionals not only to comply with legal requirements but also to exceed them, fostering environments where positive risk-taking can thrive in harmony with the imperatives of safety, respect, and compassion.

Safe Systems of Work

Safe systems of work form the backbone of any effective risk management approach in health and social care settings, creating structured environments where safety is paramount without compromising the quality and dignity of care. At their essence, these systems encompass a comprehensive set of policies, procedures, training protocols, supervision standards, and the proper use and maintenance of equipment. Together, these elements forge a coherent framework that empowers care providers to anticipate, identify, mitigate, and respond to hazards in their daily practice. The complexity of health and social care environments, with unpredictable human behaviours, diverse service user needs, and variable physical settings, necessitates that safe systems of work are both robust and flexible, embedding safety deeply across all operational aspects.

The starting point for developing a safe system of work is the formalisation of clear, accessible policies and procedures that articulate expectations and guidance for recognising and controlling risks. Such policies do not exist in isolation; they must be underpinned by current legislation and regulatory standards, including the Health and Safety at Work Act 1974, the Management of Health and Safety at Work Regulations 1999, and the Care Quality Commission's requirements.

These documents provide a legal imperative for organisations to ensure health and safety protocols are systematically developed, communicated, and followed. Importantly, policy documents clarify responsibilities across organisational hierarchies from employers, who must provide safe environments and resources, to employees, who are duty-bound to adhere to safety standards. Procedures, then, operationalise these policies into actionable steps and protocols tailored to specific tasks and settings, such as safe manual handling techniques, infection control practices, medication administration pathways, and lone-working safeguards. When alive and effective, these documents function as living tools: regularly updated through feedback loops, incident analysis, and evolving best-practice insights, rather than as static rules gathering dust.

However, policies and procedures, no matter how comprehensive, are only meaningful when those delivering care are trained adequately to interpret and implement them confidently. Training is a pivotal component of a safe system of work, serving as both an enabler and a reassurer. Effective training goes beyond generic induction sessions; it must be ongoing, specialist, and reflective of real-world challenges, integrating theoretical knowledge with practical skills. For example, training in risk assessment principles must intertwine with hands-on instruction in hazard identification, environmental scanning, and decision-making in complex scenarios. It is vital that training sessions are interactive and grounded in the actual workplace context, involving role-playing, case studies, and simulations that mirror unpredictable service user behaviours or emergency responses. This experiential element ensures that care providers develop not only competence but also the confidence to navigate uncertainty while maintaining safe working practices. Moreover, training must also foster a culture of openness and learning, encouraging staff to report near misses, errors, or emerging hazards without fear of blame or reprisal, recognising that safety thrives in a transparent and trustful environment.

Supervision acts as the connective tissue that sustains safe systems of work, ensuring that training and policies translate into daily practice and continuous improvement. Managers and team leaders must adopt visible, supportive supervisory practices that blend oversight with mentorship and constructive feedback. Supervision is not simply about checking boxes or enforcing rules; it is intrinsically about cultivating awareness, reinforcing standards, and developing professional judgement. In practice, this means observing care delivery, highlighting safe techniques, identifying deviations or gaps, and collaboratively problem-solving with staff. Through regular supervision, emerging risks that may not be immediately obvious from a procedural view, such as interpersonal dynamics, fatigue impacts, or subtle environmental changes, can be unearthed and addressed proactively. Furthermore, good supervision nurtures staff wellbeing, recognising that psychological safety is intertwined with physical safety; a supported and confident workforce is more attentive and resilient to risks. In supporting staff through supervision, managers should encourage reflective practice, inviting care providers to critically evaluate their own decision-making and to consider how risk management principles guided their actions.

The environment and equipment employed in care activities represent another critical prism through which safe systems of work are realised. Equipment must be appropriate to the task and population, regularly inspected, maintained, and used strictly in line with manufacturer and organisational guidelines. This includes everything from manual handling aids, hoists, wheelchairs, and mobility devices to personal protective equipment (PPE) such as gloves and masks. The choice and maintenance of equipment must start with the hierarchy of controls, which prioritises eliminating hazards whenever feasible, such as redesigning processes to remove risks, then substituting with less risky alternatives, applying engineering controls (like safety barriers or ergonomic adjustments), followed by administrative controls (procedures and training), and finally, PPE as a last line of defence. For example, where a challenging service user move cannot be avoided, using a mechanical hoist operated by fully trained staff, complemented by environmental adjustments and risk-aware planning, offers a safer alternative to manual handling alone. Importantly, the presence of equipment alone is insufficient; a safe system of work ensures that equipment use is seamlessly integrated within procedural and training frameworks, so that all staff understand their purpose, capabilities, and limitations. Regular audits, equipment logs, and user feedback provide ongoing assurance and inform equipment replacement or upgrades.

An essential aspect that elevates safe systems of work from static procedures to dynamic, responsive frameworks is the capacity for flexible risk management through dynamic risk assessment. Care environments are inherently fluid; service user needs can change rapidly, environmental factors vary, and unplanned incidents occur frequently. A rigid adherence to prewritten risk assessments, without adaptability, can create gaps that endanger both service users and care providers. Dynamic risk assessment requires trained staff to continually evaluate the situation as it evolves, making on-the-spot judgments to identify immediate hazards, assess their potential impact, and tailor control measures in real time. For instance, a care provider assisting a service user may notice unexpected agitation or a new environmental obstruction; applying dynamic risk assessment means recalculating risk quickly, pausing activities if necessary, adjusting equipment use, or seeking additional support. This approach empowers front-line staff to act with autonomy while still anchoring decisions in shared organisational safety principles. It demands that organisations equip staff with the confidence, training, and authority to make such assessments, as well as mechanisms for documenting and reviewing these adaptive responses to foster shared learning. Emergency situations crystallise the importance of dynamic risk assessment, as rapid decisions under pressure must balance safety imperatives with compassionate care delivery and ethical considerations.

Effective safe systems of work may also incorporate technology to augment safety. Electronic risk management systems can facilitate easier reporting, trend analysis of data, and the dissemination of updates on hazards and controls. For example, digital platforms may prompt reminders for equipment maintenance, alert supervisors to compliance gaps, or enable near-instant sharing of emergent risk information across multi-disciplinary teams. Technology also supports training through computer-based learning modules and scenario simulations, enabling flexible access to learning resources. Nonetheless, technology should be viewed as complementary rather than a panacea; the human factors of vigilance, judgement, communication, and empathy remain paramount in thriving safe systems.

Embedding a culture that values safety requires that policies, training, supervision, and equipment use are interconnected components supported by leadership commitment and staff engagement alike. Leadership must visibly champion health and safety, reinforcing its integration into organisational values, resource allocation, and performance management. This alignment fosters an environment in which staff feel both responsible for and supported in maintaining safe systems of work. Regular audits, incident investigations, and safety committees provide formal structures for monitoring effectiveness and stimulating continuous improvement. Open channels for communication across organisational levels ensure that learnings from front-line experiences shape policy evolution and training developments, closing the loop between practice and strategy.

In conclusion, safe systems of work in health and social care are multidimensional constructs that demand conscientious design and sustained investment. Through the harmonised implementation of comprehensive policies, rigourous and contextually relevant training, nurturing supervision practices, reliable and fit-for-purpose equipment, and the embracing of dynamic risk assessment, organisations can collectively build environments where safety is not an added burden but an inherent quality of everyday operations. These systems empower care providers not only to protect service users and themselves from harm but to do so while supporting autonomy, dignity, and quality of life, affirming that safety and compassionate care advance hand in hand.

Dynamic Risk Assessment

In the ever-changing landscape of health and social care, the ability to dynamically assess risk is not merely a skill but an essential component of safeguarding service users, care providers, and the wider environment. Unlike static risk assessments, which are typically conducted in controlled, predictable circumstances and rely on predefined hazards and control measures, dynamic risk assessment thrives on fluidity. It calls for real-time judgment, adaptability, and acute awareness of evolving situations that demand immediate, often complex decision-making. Dynamic risk assessment is a continuous process of scanning the environment, interpreting cues, and swiftly implementing appropriate control measures, ranging from hazard elimination to the use of personal protective equipment (PPE), all while adhering to established safe systems of work, such as policies, procedures, and training. The inherent unpredictability in health and social care settings, whether responding to an emergency, sudden change in a service user's condition, or unanticipated environmental hazards, renders this approach invaluable.

Central to the philosophy of dynamic risk assessment is recognition that conditions within care environments can transform with remarkable speed. Consider, for instance, a care provider assisting a service user with mobility who unexpectedly begins to experience breathlessness or confusion; the static risk plan might not have anticipated this scenario or provided adequate provisions. At that moment, the practitioner must evaluate emergent signs and symptoms, weigh potential risks of different actions such as calling emergency services, administering first aid, or modifying the support approach and promptly implement protective measures. This in-the-moment evaluation transcends written assessments, testing the professional's experiential knowledge, intuition, and ethical judgment. It represents an interplay of proactive vigilance and reactive agility, harmonised to ensure safety without compromising dignity or autonomy.

The foundations of this practice lie in a thorough understanding and application of control hierarchies. Dynamic risk assessment, while rapid and flexible, should systematically consider options ranging from complete hazard elimination to reliance on personal protective equipment. Elimination remains the most robust form of risk control and, when feasible, must be the immediate priority. For example, if an environmental hazard, such as a spill, is detected during a home visit, removing or containing the spill before continuing care activities mitigates danger at its source. However, in fluid situations where hazards cannot be removed immediately, substitution or engineering controls might be explored later, perhaps by employing safer alternatives or temporarily restricting access to risky zones.

Administrative controls crucially underpin dynamic responses. Well-crafted policies and procedures serve as cognitive anchors for care staff, guiding them on how to proceed in unfamiliar or pressing circumstances. These guidelines, distilled from legal and professional frameworks, instil clarity and consistency. For dynamic risk assessment to be truly effective, care organisations must invest in ongoing training that not only educates staff on standardised protocols but also hones critical-thinking skills essential for dynamic judgment. Scenario-based training, for example, simulates emergencies or complex care episodes, enabling practitioners to rehearse fluid decision-making within a safety net. Such preparation enhances confidence and capacity to assess and manage risk dynamically without undue hesitation or error. The value of good training is most evident in real crises, when prompt, confident action can literally save lives.

Personal protective equipment, while often viewed as a last resort in the control hierarchy, constitutes an indispensable line of defence when hazards cannot be fully controlled otherwise. In the face of biological threats such as infectious diseases or chemical exposures in health and social care environments, dynamic risk assessment must include the immediate selection, donning, and appropriate use of PPE to limit harm while ensuring that continuing care is delivered safely. The effective use of PPE requires not only availability and fit but also user competence and knowledge of when and how to use gloves, masks, gowns, or eye protection in response to shifting risk profiles. By integrating anticipatory planning with responsive adaptation, practitioners can fluidly incorporate PPE use into their dynamic control measures, balancing protection with practicality.

Embedding dynamic risk assessment within safe systems of work requires organisations to create a culture in which flexibility and responsiveness are valued as complementary, rather than undermining, to protocol adherence. Rigidity in policy can hinder the rapid recalibrations necessary during emergencies or unpredictable situations. Therefore, policies should articulate frameworks and principles for risk management alongside empowering practitioners to exercise professional judgment. One effective approach is to establish clear reporting and escalation pathways that accompany dynamic decisions, ensuring that when care providers deviate from prescribed measures due to emergent risk factors, such adaptations are documented, communicated, and reviewed. This transparency fosters learning, accountability, and continuous improvement in risk management.

Recognising the complex variables that challenge predictability in health and social care settings, dynamic risk assessment is inherently iterative. A practitioner may begin by identifying an immediate hazard, swiftly applying control measures, and then continually reassessing as circumstances evolve. For example, in an emergency such as a fire in a care facility, initial actions would involve fire containment and service user evacuation, while staff must simultaneously balance individual needs, mobility constraints, and potential panicked behaviour. As the situation unfolds, reassessment prompted by changing fire spread, infrastructure damage, or personnel availability is vital. This cyclical pattern of assessment and action embodies the dynamic risk assessment principle, where safety is actively "managed" rather than passively "planned."

Moreover, the human element in terms of communication, judgment, and emotional resilience is central to executing dynamic risk assessments successfully. Practitioners must maintain composure under pressure, critically assess their surroundings for new or worsening hazards, and coordinate effectively with colleagues or emergency services. Dynamic risk assessments, hence, necessitate not only technical knowledge but also emotional intelligence and interpersonal skills. During crises, clear, calm communication can mitigate panic, ensure coordinated responses, and support service users' understanding and cooperation, all of which reduce risk levels and facilitate smoother resolution.

In practice, dynamic risk assessment often manifests as mental checklists and heuristic techniques that allow practitioners to calibrate risks swiftly without extensive documentation at every moment. These cognitive tools might include evaluating the likelihood of harm in the current context, the severity of potential outcomes, and available mitigation strategies, thereby enabling pragmatic yet informed choices. While the expediency required can sometimes tempt shortcuts, it is essential that dynamic judgments remain anchored in professional standards and an ethical commitment to prioritise safety and dignity simultaneously.

To support practitioners in cultivating effective dynamic risk assessment capabilities, care organisations must integrate reflective practice into their routines. Following an incident, debriefing sessions provide invaluable opportunities to examine decisions made, discuss the effectiveness of controls deployed, and identify lessons learned. These reflective exercises reinforce learning, reveal gaps in existing procedures, and often inspire adaptations to training or policy that enhance resilience to future unexpected events. Encouraging a blame-free culture during such reflections ensures staff feel psychologically safe to share candid insights without fear, thereby promoting genuine growth and collective competence.

A significant challenge resides in balancing the competing imperatives of swift action and comprehensive documentation. While dynamic situations call for immediate intervention, the need for accurate recording cannot be sidelined, given its role in accountability, legal compliance, and quality assurance. Organisations can alleviate this tension by implementing streamlined reporting mechanisms tailored for emergencies or fast-moving scenarios, such as brief incident logs or voice-recorded reports to be transcribed later. Such innovations maintain the integrity of documentation without impeding life-saving responsiveness.

Technology also offers promising avenues to enhance dynamic risk assessments. For example, mobile devices and apps can support real-time risk evaluation by providing instant access to hazard checklists, emergency contact details, or clinical guidelines. Wearable sensors may alert to environmental dangers or physiological anomalies in service users, triggering immediate reassessment. Although technological solutions are not substitutes for human judgment, when integrated thoughtfully, they can augment situational awareness and decision-making speed, further strengthening dynamic risk management in health and social care.

Another dimension of applying dynamic risk assessment involves navigating ethical considerations inherent in rapid decision-making. Practitioners frequently face dilemmas around autonomy, consent, and acceptable risk when emerging situations demand immediate action. For instance, when a service user resists emergency intervention, the practitioner must weigh respect for their choices against the duty of care and potential harm. Dynamic risk assessment must thus incorporate ethical reasoning frameworks, ensuring that these nuanced decisions align with safeguarding principles and the individual's rights wherever possible.

Furthermore, multi-agency cooperation is paramount during complex incidents that require dynamic coordination among health, social care, emergency services, and regulatory bodies. Effective dynamic risk assessment extends beyond individual practitioners to encompass communication channels, shared protocols, and joint response plans that facilitate cohesive action despite unpredictability. Regular inter-agency drills and information sharing lay the groundwork for such collaboration, ensuring that when emergencies arise, responses are coordinated efficiently with minimised duplication or oversight.

Incorporating dynamic risk assessment into everyday practice ultimately fosters a more resilient risk culture in health and social care environments. It cultivates an ethos where staff feel empowered, equipped, and expected to respond adaptively to unexpected changes while remaining anchored in best practices and core values. When an organisation embraces this approach wholeheartedly, it strengthens its capacity not only to manage hazards in the moment but also to evolve continuously through learning, innovation, and shared experience.

To conclude, dynamic risk assessment represents a sophisticated and indispensable approach in health and social care, intertwining practical controls such as elimination, substitution, engineering controls, administrative measures, and PPE with agile judgement and ethical sensitivity. It demands constant vigilance, situational awareness, and robust training underpinned by supportive policies and systems that recognise the unpredictable nature of care delivery. By nurturing these capabilities, the sector can better protect the well-being of service users and practitioners alike, adapt to emergent challenges confidently, and ultimately advance the quality and safety of care in all settings.

Risk Assessment in Practice

Person-Centred Risk Assessment

In the complex tapestry of health and social care, person-centred risk assessment emerges not merely as a procedural task but as a profound commitment to uphold the dignity, autonomy, and individuality of service users. This approach transcends the traditional, mechanical evaluation of hazards and probabilities, calling instead for a nuanced, empathetic engagement with each person's unique circumstances, aspirations, and capacities. At the heart of person-centred risk assessment lies the delicate balance between safeguarding safety and fostering independence, a balance that requires sensitivity, respect, and genuine partnership with those receiving care.

Empowerment and choice stand as foundational pillars in this paradigm. Rather than perceiving risk as a barrier to be eliminated, person-centred assessment recognises risk as an inherent part of living, a necessary element in enabling people to exercise control over their lives. It demands an intricate understanding that while safety is paramount, protecting individuals at all costs can inadvertently strip away their opportunities for growth, dignity, and personal fulfilment. This philosophy challenges care providers to move beyond a fear-driven mindset and towards one that embraces positive risk-taking as a catalyst for empowerment. By involving service users in discussions about risk, recognising their right to make decisions, even those that may entail potential harm, professionals affirm respect for their autonomy and personhood.

This participatory approach requires transparent communication where service users are neither patronised nor shielded from the truth but are supported to understand possible outcomes and weigh options. For many, this process enhances confidence and fosters trust between care providers and service users. It also demands a commitment to ongoing dialogue, recognising that preferences and capacities may evolve, and risk assessments must be dynamic rather than static. Care providers must skilfully navigate the tensions that arise when a service user's choices appear to increase vulnerability, negotiating solutions that respect choice while ensuring reasonable protections.

Central to the enactment of person-centred risk assessment is the meticulous integration of respect for dignity throughout all interactions and decisions. Dignity is not a peripheral concern but a cornerstone that shapes how risks are identified, communicated, and managed. This means acknowledging the whole person, their history, culture, values, and relationships, and ensuring that risk management strategies do not reduce individuals to mere objects of care but honour their identity and aspirations. Even in clinical or emergency scenarios, care providers must strive to maintain privacy, seek consent when possible, and avoid actions that could cause embarrassment or disempowerment. This approach inherently challenges any paternalistic tendencies and insists on partnership, in which risks are managed with the individual rather than imposed upon them.

A crucial practical aspect of implementing person-centred risk assessment is tailoring standard risk evaluation frameworks to align with individual needs. For instance, moving and handling procedures, a common focus in care settings due to their potential to cause injury, must be adapted to empower service users. Rather than rigidly applying protocols, practitioners must assess how to support a person's movement in ways that promote independence and respect comfort, ensuring that assistive equipment or techniques enhance, rather than inhibit, autonomy. Through collaborative planning, service users can contribute insights into their capabilities and preferences, enabling care providers to balance safe practice with support for mobility.

Medication management similarly benefits from a person-centred lens. It involves not only ensuring the correct administration and monitoring for side effects but also respecting service users' rights to information, explanation, and involvement in decisions about their treatment. Encouraging autonomy in medication adherence may involve providing education, fostering self-administration skills, or developing tailored reminders, always with sensitivity to the individual's cognitive and emotional state. When risks of non-compliance or adverse reactions exist, person-centred assessment prompts practitioners to seek solutions collaboratively rather than defaulting to restrictive or coercive measures, thereby maintaining trust and dignity.

Infection control, an area intensified by global events and the constant vigilance required in care settings, presents unique challenges and opportunities for person-centred practice. Protecting individuals and communities from infection must be balanced against the risk of isolation, loss of social contact, and infringement on personal freedoms. Effective infection control strategies borne from person-centred principles involve clear, respectful communication about risks and preventive actions, incorporating service users' preferences and fostering their active participation. This could mean co-creating hygiene routines, explaining the rationale behind measures, and adjusting protocols to minimise distress or disruption, thereby reinforcing respect and empowerment even amidst necessary restrictions.

Safeguarding is a critical domain where person-centred risk assessment is indispensable. Recognising that safeguarding is not only about protection but also about preserving rights and choices reframes risk assessment from a defensive posture into an enabling practice. Care providers must approach safeguarding concerns with a mindset that seeks to listen to and amplify the voices of service users, especially those who may be vulnerable to abuse or neglect. This involves ensuring processes are transparent and trauma-informed, and that service users are active participants in decisions affecting their safety. Risk assessments here extend beyond identifying external threats to include evaluating internal vulnerabilities and strengths, and shaping interventions that are respectful and proportionate.

Lone working, often a routine yet potentially high-risk scenario in health and social care, also demands a person-centred framework. Professionals working alone must be equipped with robust risk assessments that consider their individual skills, environments, and the specific needs of those they support. For service users receiving care from lone workers, risk management must similarly account for their preferences, social context, and trust in the caregiver. Ensuring that lone working protocols include considerations of communication, emergency responses, and personal boundaries enhances safety while respecting the dignity and independence of all involved.

Embedding person-centred risk assessment across these typical care domains requires systemic commitment. It involves cultivating an organisational culture where risk is not framed solely as a hazard but as a shared responsibility, managed through collaboration, openness, and respect. Training for care providers must go beyond technical skills to develop emotional intelligence, communication competencies, and ethical reflection. This equips professionals to engage in meaningful conversations about risk and to advocate for approaches that uphold empowerment and dignity under pressure.

Moreover, documentation and reporting mechanisms must reflect the person-centred ethos. This means that records are not only factual inventories of risks and controls but also narratives that capture the person's voice, choices, and experiences. Such documentation supports continuity of care, accountability, and ongoing review, ensuring that risk assessment remains a living practice attuned to changing circumstances. It also fosters transparency with service users and their families, strengthening trust and participation.

Ultimately, person-centred risk assessment serves as a powerful antidote to reductionist models that prioritise institutional safety over individual flourishing. It aligns with contemporary health and social care values that cherish human rights, equality, and personhood. Despite the complexity and challenges inherent in balancing risk and independence, this approach offers a hopeful vision where safety and dignity coexist harmoniously, enabling people to lead meaningful lives supported by confident, compassionate care providers. It is a dynamic, relational process that honours the diversity of human experience and affirms the fundamental principle that care is at its best when it sees and respects the whole person.

Common Risk Assessments in Care

In the intricate and dynamic setting of health and social care, certain types of risk assessments are consistently encountered due to the nature of the work and the vulnerabilities of the individuals involved. These common risk assessments not only serve as foundational pillars in maintaining safety but also are crucial in supporting the delicate balance between managing risks and promoting autonomy, dignity, and independence for service users. Each of these assessments embodies unique challenges, encompassing technical procedures, ethical considerations, and the imperative of person-centred care. An in-depth exploration of these common risk assessments, covering moving and handling, medication management, infection control, safeguarding, and lone working, illuminates their pivotal role in fostering safe, respectful, and empowering care environments.

Moving and handling risk assessments are vital components in care settings where physical assistance is frequently necessary. The act of moving or repositioning service users, whether it involves transferring from a bed to a wheelchair or supporting mobility during activities, inherently carries significant risk to both the care provider and the service user. The physical demands on carers can lead to musculoskeletal injuries, often culminating in long-term absence and compromised workforce capability, while improper handling risks falls, bruising, fractures, or pain for the recipient of care. The process of conducting these risk assessments entails a comprehensive understanding of both the physical environment and the individual's abilities, needs, and preferences. Care providers must consider factors such as the service user's level of strength, balance, and cognitive function, alongside an appraisal of the available equipment, space, and staff support. More abstractly, this assessment must be attuned to the importance of preserving the service user's dignity and independence. Often, a fine line exists between necessary assistance and undue restriction, and the risk assessment must navigate this sensitively. For example, encouraging service users to participate actively in their own movement, wherever feasible, not only mitigates risk but also dignifies and empowers them. This promotes a person-centred approach in which care is tailored to individual capabilities and preferences rather than a one-size-fits-all approach. The risk assessment, therefore, transcends mere compliance, becoming an opportunity to engage users meaningfully in decision-making about their care. Enhanced by practical tools such as mechanical aids, hoists, slide sheets, or transfer boards, the assessment weighs the benefits of these interventions against the potential discomfort or loss of autonomy they may entail. Collaboration with physiotherapists or occupational therapists often enriches this process, bringing expert insight to optimise safety and independence. Importantly, the risk assessment is not static but requires ongoing evaluation as the service user's condition evolves. The documentation of these assessments, coupled with staff training in safe techniques, reinforces a culture of safety and respect.

Medication risk assessments present a complex domain where precision, vigilance, and empathy converge. Medicines form a cornerstone of health management, yet the administration, storage, and monitoring of medication carry multiple layers of risk from adverse reactions and interactions to errors stemming from miscommunication or lapses in protocols. Comprehensive medication risk assessment involves a meticulous examination of the individual's prescriptions, the suitability and timing of dosages, potential contraindications, and the service user's capacity to self-administer or understand medication instructions. It further requires consideration of external factors, such as the configuration of storage facilities and the availability of support tools, such as pill organisers or reminders. Beyond logistics, this assessment is intricately tied to respecting autonomy, as many service users prefer to retain control over their medication routines. The assessment must capture this preference and weigh it against safety imperatives. Collaborative conversations amongst care providers, pharmacists, and the service user, sometimes extended to family or advocates, are crucial to navigate these tensions. Equally, the assessment acknowledges the emotional impact medication regimes may have, such as anxiety about side effects or the stigma associated with certain prescriptions. By fostering an open, person-centred dialogue alongside the technical assessment of safety, care providers can tailor support plans that uphold independence without compromising well-being. Environmental variables, such as ensuring medicines are stored at the correct temperatures and protected from unauthorised access, are integrated into the risk judgment, alongside scheduled reviews to detect any adverse developments promptly. The inclusion of structured medication administration records, double-checking procedures, and staff training fortifies the framework within which these assessments operate. In essence, medication risk assessments serve as a fulcrum balancing the clinical rigour of pharmaceutical safety with the humane respect for individual choice and trust.

Infection control risk assessments have gained universal prominence, given the ever-present threat of infectious diseases in communal health and social care settings. The challenge extends beyond preventing microbial transmission to encompass safeguarding the psychological comfort and personal integrity of service users. Deliberate and strategic infection control is particularly critical among populations who may have compromised immune systems, chronic conditions, or limited ability to advocate for themselves. The assessment undertakes a thorough analysis of the environment, including cleanliness, sanitisation protocols, availability of handwashing facilities, and use of personal protective equipment, paired with the evaluation of routine practices such as waste disposal and laundry handling. Furthermore, it evaluates the behaviours of staff, visitors, and service users to ensure compliance with established guidelines and to identify gaps or potential sources of contamination. Integral to this process is education: ensuring that all stakeholders understand the rationale behind infection control measures fosters cooperation and reduces resistance. From a dignity perspective, infection control measures may sometimes appear restrictive or isolating. For instance, the need for quarantine or isolation might conflict with a service user's desire for social interaction, presenting a tension that the risk assessment must navigate with sensitivity. Equally, the use of protective gear can inadvertently depersonalise interactions, posing a challenge to empathetic care. The skilful crafting of this risk assessment involves embedding infection prevention within a framework of respect and communication, explaining the necessity of measures in an accessible language, and involving service users in decisions to the extent possible. Importantly, infection control is a field subject to rapid changes in knowledge, as witnessed during global health crises like the COVID-19 pandemic, which demand that risk assessments be both robust and adaptable. Regular audits, environmental monitoring, and incident reporting mechanisms form part of an active risk management culture. Within this, the assessment is not a checkbox exercise but a living document that reflects current best practice, staff training levels, and evolving public health guidance. Its success lies in balancing rigourous scientific standards with a compassionate approach that respects human needs and dignity.

Safeguarding risk assessments form a critical refuge in health and social care, designed to protect individuals from abuse, neglect, and exploitation. The complexity of safeguarding arises from its foundation in human rights, ethics, and the protection of vulnerability, making the associated risk assessments not only technical but profoundly relational and moral undertakings. These assessments require acute awareness of risk factors within the interpersonal dynamics among service users, care providers, family members, and wider networks. Safeguarding risk assessments extend beyond obvious physical threats to include emotional, financial, or institutional abuse, acknowledging the diversity of potential harm. The process begins with vigilant observation, active listening, and consistent questioning, paired with thorough documentation and multi-agency collaboration when concerns arise. Crucially, the assessment must be sensitive to power imbalances and the potential for discrimination or bias within care systems themselves. Respecting the service user's voice and autonomy is imperative here, even when making difficult decisions that restrict freedom to enhance safety. The assessment balances these competing priorities through careful analysis, ensuring that protective actions do not inadvertently contribute to disempowerment or stigmatisation. Understanding cultural contexts, personal histories, and psychological factors enriches the risk evaluation and response. Training for staff on recognising and reporting safeguarding concerns is vital, as is creating an environment that supports whistleblowing and ensures concerns are acted upon promptly. Establishing clear escalation pathways ensures that identified risks are addressed in a timely manner and with appropriate expertise, involving social services, healthcare professionals, or regulatory agencies as necessary. Fundamentally, safeguarding risk assessments act as a moral compass within care, guiding not only procedural adherence but also the upholding of human dignity and justice. They are not static but evolve with changing circumstances, necessitating continuous reassessment and collaboration.

Lone working risk assessments address the unique challenges presented when care providers operate independently, often isolated from immediate support and in varied environments. Lone working is common in domiciliary care, community nursing, and outreach roles, where unpredictability and vulnerability to hazards are heightened. These assessments systematically analyse the physical risks of the setting, including access points, environmental hazards, and security measures, as well as the procedural risks related to communication, emergency response, and workload management. Key to this assessment is the consideration of personal safety, ensuring that staff have effective means of summoning help if needed and that risk factors associated with specific service users, such as aggressive behaviours or complex needs, are thoroughly evaluated and mitigated. The emotional and psychological impact of lone working must not be underestimated; feelings of isolation or stress can affect decision-making and overall well-being. From a service user perspective, ensuring that lone working does not compromise their needs for safe, consistent care is integral. The assessment must weigh these dual perspectives, often involving service user input, to understand how visits and interactions can be structured to minimise risk without diminishing relationship quality or responsiveness. Technological aids, such as personal alarms, mobile phones with GPS tracking, and robust scheduling systems, are incorporated as strategies within the risk management process. Training on assertiveness, conflict resolution, and self-care also forms part of a comprehensive approach. The recording of risk assessments includes contingency plans outlining actions in emergencies, communication protocols, and follow-up procedures. Organisations foster cultures that support lone workers through regular check-ins, supervision, and forums for feedback, embedding the assessment into a living framework of support and accountability. Ensuring that lone working assessments are dynamic and sensitive to contextual changes, be they environmental, personal, or organisational, is crucial for sustaining both staff safety and quality of care.

Across all these common risk assessments, a unifying thread is the essential need to balance the innate risks involved in care with the empowerment of service users and the maintenance of dignity. This balance resists a simplistic risk-averse mentality that might lead to overly restrictive or paternalistic care models, instead championing "positive risk-taking." Positive risk-taking recognises that absolute safety is neither possible nor desirable; rather, some risks are necessary for growth, independence, and quality of life. In practical terms, this means involving service users as active participants in their risk assessments, consulting them, respecting their preferences, and jointly formulating strategies that enable informed choices. This approach calls for transparent communication and mutual trust, allowing care providers to negotiate safety boundaries without undermining autonomy. Documentation and policies that embed person-centred language and frameworks reinforce this ethos.

Additionally, maintaining dignity throughout risk assessment processes requires sensitivity to individuals' cultural backgrounds, values, and past experiences. Care providers who invest time in building genuine relationships foster environments where discussions of risk can be open and non-threatening. This transparency increases the accuracy and effectiveness of assessments, as service users are more likely to disclose fears or preferences. In some cases, specialised advocacy or peer support enhances this dialogue.

While technical competence is crucial for each specific type of risk assessment, the holistic view must integrate these assessments into the broader context of care planning. For instance, moving and handling risks often intersect with medication side effects affecting mobility, with safeguarding concerns related to dependency and autonomy. Infection control strategies have implications for the environment in which lone working takes place, affecting security and emergency readiness. Recognising these intersections fosters more coherent, comprehensive risk management that transcends fragmented approaches.

Ultimately, common risk assessments in health and social care are living, evolving entities shaped by the interplay of clinical evidence, ethical principles, human relationships, and organisational cultures. Their effectiveness hinges on care providers' commitment to view risk assessment not as an administrative hurdle but as a dynamic, person-centred practice essential to quality care. Through continuous learning, respectful engagement with service users, and reflective practice, care professionals transform risk assessments from abstract instruments into empowering tools that safeguard health, uphold dignity, and promote independence in meaningful ways.

Recording, Reporting, and Reviewing

Documentation

Effective documentation stands as the cornerstone of sound risk assessment practice in health and social care, binding together the myriad actions, decisions, and reflections that underpin the commitment to safeguarding both service users and care providers. The complexity and dynamism of care environments necessitate a robust, meticulous approach to recording risk-related information, which serves not only as a legal and regulatory safeguard but also as an essential tool for communication, learning, and continuous improvement within the care setting. It is within these written records, spanning risk assessment forms, care plans, and incident and accident reports, that the nuances and realities of risk management are captured, analysed, and responded to. This documentation, far from being a mere bureaucratic exercise, forms the living archive of care quality and safety.

Risk assessment forms are among the primary documents in this landscape, serving as structured frameworks for identifying hazards, evaluating risks, and determining appropriate control measures. These forms are meticulously designed to guide practitioners through a systematic process, first prompting the clear identification of potential hazards within specific care scenarios or environments. From physical risks such as slippery floors or faulty equipment to psychological risks like stress or neglect, every conceivable hazard must be captured with precision. The forms then guide the assessor in analysing these risks by considering the likelihood of occurrence and the potential severity of impact, often using risk matrices or scoring systems. This analytical step ensures that responses are proportionate and prioritised effectively. Crucially, risk assessment forms do not end with identification and analysis; they also include detailed records of planned control measures, responsible persons for implementation, and review timelines. This ensures ownership and accountability within the team. Moreover, contemporary forms frequently include prompts to consider service users' perspectives and rights, reflecting the broader ethos of empowerment and person-centred care. The dynamic nature of care demands that these risk assessments be revisited regularly, at intervals dictated by the evolving risk landscape or following any relevant incidents, ensuring that safeguards remain responsive and effective.

Complementing risk assessment forms, care plans play an indispensable role in embedding risk management into the daily reality of service delivery. Unlike the more general, environmental focus of risk assessment forms, care plans translate risk considerations into personalised strategies that acknowledge everyone's unique circumstances, preferences, and capabilities. The process of developing a care plan involves synthesising information from the risk assessment alongside detailed knowledge of the service user's health status, lifestyle, goals, and support networks. Within the care plan, identified risks are balanced against the imperative to promote independence and dignity, illustrating the nuanced philosophy of positive risk-taking. Documentation within the care plan clearly outlines agreed goals, tailored support measures, and precautionary steps that both protect and empower the individual. This might include, for example, positioning aids for a service user with mobility issues to prevent falls, alongside explicit encouragement and assistance plans that foster confidence in movement. The care plan thus becomes a living document, referenced and adjusted through daily practice, multidisciplinary collaboration, and ongoing dialogue with the service user. Meticulous documentation here serves a dual purpose: it ensures continuity and consistency of care across shifts and disciplines, and it provides an evidential record that protections and freedoms have been considered and communicated transparently.

Integral to the ecosystem of documentation are incident and accident reports, which provide crucial retrospective insights into risk events when controls fail or unforeseen circumstances arise. These reports serve as formal records that detail the nature, context, and consequences of incidents ranging from minor injuries to near misses and significant adverse events. The precision and completeness of these reports are vital. They typically require a factual, unbiased account, including the date, time, location, persons involved, and a thorough description of what occurred. Importantly, these narratives must move beyond surface descriptions to analyse contributory factors such as the equipment being faulty, whether supervision was inadequate, or whether there were unexpected changes in the environment. This level of detail enables organisations to identify systemic weaknesses or emerging hazards before they precipitate further harm. Additionally, incident reports form the foundation for reflective practice and learning, triggering reviews of existing risk assessments, care plans, or procedural safeguards. Timely and accurate completion of these reports is paramount, and health and social care organisations often have stringent policies mandating prompt documentation to preserve detail reliability and enable swift response.

Reporting procedures extend beyond internal documentation, encompassing obligations to regulatory bodies and legal frameworks, which amplify the significance of diligent recording and transparency. The importance of whistleblowing mechanisms cannot be overstated in this context; they offer professionals a confidential and protected avenue to report concerns about unsafe practices, neglect, or breaches of duty when internal procedures may be compromised or ignored. Encouraging a culture where staff feel confident and supported to raise such concerns fortifies the overall safety architecture. Parallelly, adherence to statutory requirements such as the Reporting of Injuries, Diseases and Dangerous Occurrences Regulations 2013 (RIDDOR) in the UK mandates that certain incidents, specifically those involving serious injuries, fatalities, occupational diseases, or dangerous occurrences, are reported promptly to the Health and Safety Executive (HSE). The documentation associated with RIDDOR reporting must be precise, comprehensive, and comply with designated timeframes to ensure legal compliance and enable regulatory oversight. Not only does this legal obligation drive improvements in workplace safety through statistical monitoring and intervention, but it also reinforces organisational accountability. For care providers, understanding which events trigger RIDDOR, how to document them properly, and the subsequent steps following such reporting is essential knowledge embedded within organisational training and policies.

Regular review and updating of all risk-related documentation underpin a culture of continuous improvement rather than complacency. Risk assessment forms and care plans are not static artefacts; they are living documents demanding periodic reassessment at scheduled intervals or in response to changes, such as new medications, revised care settings, or emerging health conditions. The act of reviewing serves several pivotal functions: it verifies that control measures remain effective, assesses whether risk levels have shifted, and integrates new information gathered through ongoing monitoring or incident analysis. Documentation of these reviews must be thorough, capturing not only any amendments made but also rationales for changes or decisions to maintain existing strategies. The cyclical nature of documentation, from initial assessment through to review and revision, reflects the dynamic and responsive ethos vital to the health and social care sector. This ensures that risk management stays aligned with the evolving needs of service users and the practical realities of care delivery.

Furthermore, effective documentation enhances communication across all levels of the care team and with external agencies. Accurate and accessible records enable frontline care providers, managers, and regulatory agents to share a common understanding of risk profiles and control strategies. This collective awareness fosters coordinated action, reduces duplication or contradiction of efforts, and supports transparent dialogue with service users and their families. Furthermore, well-maintained documentation is invaluable during inspections, audits, and quality assurance processes, where evidence of diligent risk management and compliance is scrutinised. From the perspective of service users, accessible documentation that is explained in plain language strengthens trust and inclusion, empowering individuals to participate in discussions about their safety and risk tolerance.

In sum, the careful crafting, management, and review of documentation are not peripheral tasks but central pillars of effective risk assessment in health and social care. Through risk assessment forms, care plans, incident and accident reports, and formal regulatory submissions, documentation weaves a narrative of vigilance, accountability, and compassion. It enables care providers to translate abstract concepts of risk into concrete protective actions, while simultaneously honouring the rights and dignity of those they serve. Committing to high standards of documentation is a commitment to excellence in care, one that promotes safety, supports independence, encourages transparency, and fosters a culture of learning and improvement that benefits all stakeholders in the health and social care environment.

Reporting Procedures

Effective reporting procedures form the backbone of a safe and compliant health and social care environment, functioning as both a protective shield for those who provide and receive care and as a critical mechanism for organisational learning and continuous improvement. Within this complex system, understanding the full spectrum of reporting from frontline incident documentation to whistleblowing and statutory notifications such as those required by RIDDOR (Reporting of Injuries, Diseases and Dangerous Occurrences Regulations) is imperative. Each facet plays a significant role in embedding a culture of openness, accountability, and proactive risk management. The seamless integration of these reporting mechanisms ensures that risks are identified promptly, incidents are managed correctly, and lessons learned translate into better care outcomes and the safeguarding of all involved.

At its core, the reporting process begins with accurate and timely documentation. This is not merely a bureaucratic formality but a vital communication tool that ensures essential information about incidents, near misses, or hazards reaches the appropriate individuals and authorities. The nature and depth of documentation must reflect the complexity of the incident and its impact on service users and staff. Whether it involves a minor slip within a care home or a more severe safeguarding concern, precise details must be recorded, including the circumstances surrounding the event, the people involved, the immediate measures taken, and any subsequent actions planned. These records serve multiple purposes: they provide a legal audit trail, support investigations or inquiries, and feed into risk assessments that allow preventative strategies to evolve.

Escalation processes are the lifeline that thread through the reporting system, defining how and when information moves up the hierarchy to those with the authority and responsibility to intervene. In health and social care settings, this escalation is not a rigid, one-size-fits-all journey but a flexible pathway governed by the severity and urgency of the issue. Minor concerns may be resolved at the team level through informal discussions or adjustments, yet more serious incidents demand formal notification to managers or specialist teams, such as safeguarding leads or health and safety officers. Clarity in escalation pathways is essential; everyone within the organisation must understand their role in raising concerns and the channels available for doing so. This clarity helps prevent delays in responses that could exacerbate harm or allow unsafe conditions to persist. It also underscores a culture in which raising a concern is seen as a positive contribution to workplace safety and quality care, rather than a cause for blame or retribution.

Within the realm of escalation lies the critical area of whistleblowing, a process that empowers care workers and professionals to expose wrongdoing or serious risks without fear of reprisal. Whistleblowing acts as a safety net for revealing issues that may not be picked up through normal reporting lines or that involve those in positions of authority. In health and social care, where vulnerable individuals depend heavily on practitioners, whistleblowing is both an ethical imperative and a legal right, enshrined in the Public Interest Disclosure Act 1998. It allows professionals to speak out about malpractice, neglect, abuse, or systemic failures that compromise standards of care. For whistleblowing to be effective, care organisations must cultivate an environment of trust and transparency in which staff know that raising concerns is protected and valued. This includes clear policies, confidential reporting mechanisms, and assurances against victimisation. Training and awareness campaigns about whistleblowing rights and responsibilities further strengthen this culture. When whistleblowers are supported, the organisation benefits not only from resolving immediate problems but also from preventing future risks and reinforcing a commitment to best practice.

Parallel to internal reporting structures, statutory reporting is a distinct yet fully integrated requirement that health and social care providers must adhere to in alignment with UK legislation. The RIDDOR framework exemplifies such a statutory obligation, under which organisations must report to the Health and Safety Executive (HSE) fatal injuries, major incidents, certain work-related illnesses, and dangerous occurrences in the workplace. These reports enable regulatory authorities to monitor safety standards, investigate causes, and, where necessary, enforce compliance or prosecute negligence. RIDDOR demands specific criteria for reporting, strict timeframes, and designated persons, usually managers or health and safety leads, to take responsibility for submitting reports. Failure to comply can result in significant legal consequences, reputational damage, and, more importantly, ongoing hazards that might threaten life or health. Beyond RIDDOR, care organisations might also be obliged to notify other bodies, such as the Care Quality Commission (CQC), in cases of safeguarding incidents or persistent service failures. Familiarity with all relevant statutory reporting requirements and mechanisms is therefore vital and forms a key dimension of effective risk management.

Documenting and reporting are only as effective as the feedback loops and review mechanisms built around them. Regular reviews of incident reports and risk assessments allow care providers to detect patterns or recurring issues that may not be apparent from isolated events. These reviews should be conducted systematically, involving multidisciplinary teams where appropriate, to scrutinise causes, evaluate the effectiveness of controls implemented, and identify opportunities for improvement. Reflections informed by comprehensive data feed into organisational learning, underpin continuous professional development, and align with external audit and inspection regimes. For example, trends in medication errors reported through documentation and subsequent audits can lead to enhanced training programs, redesigned protocols, or technological supports such as electronic prescribing systems. Cognisant that health and social care environments are dynamic, reviews must also accommodate emerging risks arising from changes in service user profiles, new therapies, or environmental factors such as outbreaks of infection.

The quality of reporting documentation itself is a cornerstone of the entire system. Poorly completed, vague, or delayed reports can negate the benefits of reporting mechanisms. Therefore, organisations invest in training care staff not only on the 'what' and 'when' to report but critically on the 'how' the clarity, accuracy, and objectivity required in their documentation. Clear language, avoidance of jargon, factual rather than emotional descriptions, and confidentiality considerations all contribute to the integrity and utility of reports. Digital record-keeping, increasingly prevalent across care settings, offers advantages for accessibility, analysis, and storage but must be balanced with secure data protection practices. Written reports also serve as vital evidence in legal or regulatory inquiries; hence, attention to detail upholds professional standards and safeguards organisational interests.

Whistleblowing, while often viewed as a last resort or an isolated act, is better understood as part of a continuum of reporting that begins with open dialogue and clear internal communication. In environments where staff feel psychologically safe to voice concerns without stigma or retaliation, problems are often resolved before they escalate to formal whistleblowing or statutory notification. Leadership styles anchored in transparency, respect, and responsiveness form the bedrock of this culture. Senior managers are tasked with modelling openness, promptly addressing issues raised, and ensuring that feedback is not only given but also visibly acted upon. This responsiveness reassures staff that their contributions genuinely influence the quality and safety of care, reinforcing morale and commitment. Where whistleblowing does become necessary, support mechanisms such as access to independent advice lines, trade unions, or regulatory bodies complement internal policies and form a wider safety net.

Moreover, escalation and reporting must navigate the delicate balance between organisational accountability and individual privacy. In health and social care, the handling of incident and risk information involves sensitive personal data about service users and staff, invoking data protection laws such as the General Data Protection Regulation (GDPR). Reporting procedures must therefore embed sound confidentiality practices to protect identities while ensuring that necessary information flows unimpeded to those responsible for managing risk. This balancing act requires clear internal guidance on who can access reports, how data is anonymised when shared, and protocols for sharing information with external agencies. These considerations extend to whistleblowing cases where confidentiality and anonymity arc paramount to protect the reporter. Ethical handling of data within reporting systems fosters trust, maximises cooperation, and complies with legal obligations.

The reporting system, taken as a whole, is not static but evolves continuously through feedback and learning. Organisations that succeed in this evolution create formal mechanisms for debriefing after incidents and incorporate lessons learned into policies and practice. Among these mechanisms are incident review panels, mortality and morbidity meetings, or safeguarding forums, where multidisciplinary teams analyse cases to extract actionable insights. The openness to critique and change underpins a resilient culture that treats human error as an opportunity for improvement rather than a source of blame. Such cultures encourage innovation in risk control measures and adapt rapidly to changing service environments, whether responding to new public health challenges or emerging social care needs.

While the book's scope is firmly UK-based, it is worth noting that global health and social care trends increasingly emphasise the importance of transparent, prompt, and effective reporting as a universal standard. International models highlight how robust reporting frameworks support broader public health efforts by providing data for epidemiological studies, identifying systemic vulnerabilities, and aiding resource allocation. These global perspectives further reinforce the imperative for health and social care providers to master not only local statutory requirements but also best practices in reporting and escalation as part of their professional competence.

In summary, the fabric of safe and high-quality health and social care is inseparable from the rigour, clarity, and responsiveness of its reporting procedures. From everyday documentation to whistleblowing and compliance with statutory reporting regimes, the processes in place determine an organisation's capacity to protect, learn, and improve. Integral to this is the continual review and reflection that turns reports into practical changes, enhancing care environments for service users and empowering care providers with confidence and clarity. As such, mastery of reporting protocols is not an administrative burden but a vital professional skill, an ethical responsibility, and a cornerstone of compassionate, safe care.

Reviewing Risk Assessments

Risk assessments in health and social care environments are not static documents; they are living tools designed to capture the dynamic, ever-evolving nature of care settings. The practice of reviewing risk assessments is fundamental to ensuring that the safety measures in place remain effective and relevant to the current circumstances of service users, staff, and the environment itself. A risk assessment completed once and then quickly forgotten becomes obsolete, potentially exposing individuals to unforeseen hazards or causing them to miss opportunities to support positive risk-taking and greater independence. Therefore, it is essential that health and social care professionals adopt a proactive, systematic approach to reviewing risk assessments to uphold the highest standards of safety and quality of care.

The process of reviewing risk assessments must be embedded within the routine operations of any care setting. Reviews should occur at predetermined intervals, such as monthly, quarterly, or annually, depending on the nature of the risks involved and the vulnerability of the client group. However, fixed schedules alone do not suffice. A more agile approach is required, one that triggers immediate reassessment in response to specific events or changes. For example, any incident or near-miss involving harm or potential harm mandates a prompt review. Similarly, significant changes in a service user's health status, environment, or care plan also necessitate reassessment. A newly diagnosed condition that affects mobility or cognition can dramatically alter the risk profile, necessitating a swift revision of existing control measures. The goal is to maintain an accurate picture of risks over time, avoiding complacency that can erode the quality and efficacy of risk management practices.

Effective review begins with a meticulous examination of the documentation initially created during the risk assessment process. Documentation is a cornerstone of accountability, transparency, and continuous learning. In health and social care, multiple forms of records are maintained to capture various elements of care and safety. These include written risk assessments, incident logs, safeguarding reports, service user feedback forms, and care plans. Each of these documents provides unique insights into the risks at hand and the effectiveness of existing controls. When reviewing risk assessments, practitioners must consider the entire documentation, cross-referencing details to identify emergent patterns or discrepancies. For instance, an incident log might reveal recurring slips in a particular area of a care home, prompting a physical review and potential reconfiguration of that space to mitigate risk. Similarly, feedback from service users might highlight concerns that were previously overlooked, such as the drawbacks of certain restraint techniques or challenges with medication schedules. The richness of the documentation allows for a holistic and nuanced review, moving beyond perfunctory checklist exercises to meaningful risk management.

Reporting mechanisms play a pivotal role in facilitating timely and transparent risk assessment reviews. Staff should be encouraged and supported to report incidents, near misses, and unsafe conditions without fear of blame or reprisal. The establishment of a positive reporting culture is critical; it promotes openness, learning, and early intervention. Within this framework, whistleblowing emerges as a vital safeguard, providing an avenue for raising serious concerns about unsafe practices or systemic issues that may not be adequately addressed through routine channels. Whistleblowing policies must be clearly communicated, easily accessible, and rigorously upheld to protect reporters from retaliation and to maintain the integrity of the risk management system. When a whistleblower raises concerns, these must trigger an urgent and thorough review of related risk assessments, ensuring that any underlying hazards are swiftly identified and controlled.

The legal obligations surrounding reporting and review extend beyond internal organisational policies. In the United Kingdom, care providers are bound by statutory requirements, such as the Reporting of Injuries, Diseases and Dangerous Occurrences Regulations 2013 (RIDDOR). Under RIDDOR, incidents resulting in death, specified injuries, diseases, or dangerous occurrences must be formally reported to the Health and Safety Executive (HSE). These legal mandates compel organisations to maintain meticulous records and to conduct rigorous investigations and reviews following reportable events. The process serves a dual purpose: protecting those affected and contributing to broader public health and safety data that inform sector-wide improvements. Compliance with such regulations is a protective shield against legal liability and reputational damage, and it underscores the seriousness of risk assessment as a continual, responsive activity.

In practical terms, the review of risk assessments involves revisiting the initial hazard identification and risk evaluation stages with fresh eyes and updated information. This re-examination should assess whether previously identified hazards have been effectively controlled, whether new hazards have emerged, and whether risk ratings remain valid. Reviewing the effectiveness of control measures is particularly crucial, as some interventions may lose efficacy over time or require adaptation to evolving circumstances. For example, engineering controls like handrails or emergency lighting require routine maintenance checks to ensure proper functioning. Administrative controls, such as shift patterns or training programs, may need to be adjusted to reflect changes in personnel or workload. Personal protective equipment (PPE) availability and usage also warrant reassessment as new guidance or products become available or if supply issues arise.

Beyond compliance and safety, the review process offers a valuable opportunity for reflection and learning. Care teams should engage collaboratively in this process, drawing on the diverse perspectives of managers, frontline staff, service users, and regulatory agents. Such involvement fosters a shared understanding of risks and reinforces individual accountability. It also encourages a culture of positive risk-taking, where safeguarding and empowerment are balanced thoughtfully, and where service users' voices contribute meaningfully to decisions affecting their lives. Regular training and refresher sessions can bolster the skills needed to conduct effective reviews, equip staff to interpret data and documentation critically, and inspire confidence in making responsive adjustments to care plans.

The communication of revised risk assessments is as essential as their review. Once updated, revised assessments must be disseminated promptly to all relevant parties to ensure that changes in risk status and control measures are understood and implemented. Failure to communicate alterations can result in outdated practices continuing unchecked, negating the benefits of the review. This communication can take various forms, including formal meetings, written notices, electronic systems, or one-on-one discussions, tailored to the context and complexity of the changes. Ensuring that documentation reflects the most current version of risk assessments, with clear version control and audit trails, supports transparency and accountability.

Periodic reviews may reveal broader systemic issues that require escalation beyond the immediate care setting. In such instances, multi-agency collaboration becomes vital, bringing together health and social care professionals, regulatory bodies, safeguarding teams, and sometimes law enforcement or legal advisors. Collective expertise supports the comprehensive evaluation and resolution of complex risks, such as safeguarding concerns, service-user exploitation, or environmental hazards affecting multiple sites. These partnerships exemplify best practices in risk governance and reinforce a consistent, unified approach to safety and quality.

In conclusion, the review of risk assessments is a multifaceted process demanding vigilance, diligence, and a proactive mindset. It requires attention to timing, embracing both routine and event-driven reviews, alongside scrupulous use of documentation and reporting channels. The importance of fostering a culture that values transparency, learning, and positive risk management cannot be overstated. Through committed and collaborative review practices, health and social care professionals can ensure that risk assessments remain dynamic instruments that protect and empower all stakeholders, thereby advancing the overarching mission of delivering safe, dignified, and effective care.

Promoting a Positive Risk Culture

Positive Risk-Taking

Positive risk-taking within health and social care is a profoundly pivotal concept that challenges traditional, risk-averse attitudes by advocating for empowerment and independence as fundamental rights of every service user. At its core, positive risk-taking is about recognising that absolute safety free from all risk is neither achievable nor desirable in the context of human autonomy and dignity. Instead, it embraces the notion that people, even those with vulnerabilities or complex care needs, have the right to make choices that involve risk, so long as these choices are informed, considered, and supported. This paradigm shift moves away from the old-fashioned, paternalistic approach that seeks to shield individuals from every possible danger, often at the expense of their freedom, growth, and well-being. In health and social care, positive risk-taking requires professionals to carefully balance the potential benefits and harms of any decision or action, thereby promoting independence while remaining vigilant about safeguarding concerns.

Taking a deep dive into the empowerment aspect of positive risk-taking, it is essential to understand that empowerment is not merely about granting permission to take risks but is a complex process involving information sharing, dialogue, and mutual respect. Service users must be supported in understanding the nature of the risks involved in their choices and in weighing them against their personal goals, preferences, and values. For many people, the opportunity to take on managed risks, such as engaging in social activities, making decisions about their care, or trying new therapies, can lead to enhanced self-esteem, improved mental health, and a stronger sense of control over their lives. This holistic empowerment, therefore, plays a crucial role not only in safeguarding physical safety but also in nurturing psychological and emotional well-being. It acknowledges people's right to make mistakes, recognising that learning from errors is a vital part of human development.

However, this commitment to empowerment is firmly rooted in ethical considerations that health and social care professionals must navigate with skill. Ethical dilemmas often arise when service users make choices that expose them to greater risk, such as choosing to live independently despite the risks associated with falls or medication management. Professionals can find themselves caught between the duty of care, which demands preventing harm, and the respect for autonomy, which requires honouring individuals' decisions. Resolving these tensions necessitates a sensitive, person-centred approach grounded in ethical frameworks such as beneficence, non-maleficence, autonomy, and justice. Beneficence urges care providers to act in the best interests of service users, while non-maleficence emphasises avoiding harm. Balancing these sometimes-conflicting principles with respect for autonomy calls for dialogue, negotiation, and transparent decision-making processes.

Integral to this ethical practice is the rigorous application of person-centred risk assessments that consider not only the likelihood and severity of harm but also the person's capacity to understand, consent, and adapt to risk. This assessment is not a one-off event but an ongoing conversation involving the care provider, the service user, families, and, where appropriate, advocates or legal guardians. Successfully supporting positive risk-taking demands trust and rapport, encouraging service users to voice their concerns, preferences, and goals openly. It also requires meticulous documentation to ensure that decisions are traceable, accountable, and aligned with professional standards and legal requirements.

Recognising abuse and neglect within this landscape is another critical piece of the puzzle. Positive risk-taking should never become a cover for systemic failures or inadequate safeguarding. Professionals must remain vigilant to signs that a service user may be suffering harm, whether deliberate or through neglect, while conscientiously distinguishing between genuine risks embraced by the person's informed choice and those arising from coercion, exploitation, or unsafe practices. The subtle boundaries between allowing risk and preventing harm demand a high level of professional skill and ethical judgment. Training in recognising indicators of abuse, such as unexplained injuries, withdrawal, changes in behaviour, or inconsistent explanations, is essential to ensure that empowerment is not mistaken for tolerance of preventable harm.

Effective safeguarding in the context of positive risk-taking involves nuanced, tailored interventions rather than blanket prohibitions. This requires creating safeguarding plans that incorporate the individual's voice and prioritise their preferred outcomes, even when these include certain levels of risk. It also mandates the creation of an environment in which service users feel safe reporting concerns without fear of retribution or loss of independence. This places a heavy responsibility on care providers and managers to foster a culture of openness, respect, and vigilance, in which safeguarding measures are proactive, proportionate, and embedded in routine practice rather than reactive or punitive.

Collaboration across agencies is another indispensable dimension of fostering positive risk-taking while ensuring safety. Health and social care rarely operate in silos; the complex needs of service users often require integrating input from social workers, healthcare professionals, housing providers, law enforcement, advocacy organisations, and family members. This collaborative working enhances the quality of risk management by pooling expertise, sharing information, and ensuring a consistent approach, ultimately benefiting service users through more coherent, effective support. For instance, a decision about supporting an individual with learning disabilities to participate in community activities may involve a nurse's assessment of physical risks, safeguarding reviews by a social worker, and input from community organisations to ensure accessibility and safety. Such multi-agency cooperation reinforces the principle that positive risk-taking is not reckless but managed through informed, collective responsibility.

Moreover, multi-agency collaboration serves as a safeguard against fragmented care and enables dynamic risk assessments that adapt promptly to changing circumstances or emerging threats. It facilitates a holistic understanding by combining perspectives that a single provider might overlook. However, this collaboration also requires careful navigation of confidentiality, data protection laws, and professional boundaries. Open communication channels, clear protocols, and shared training sessions can help foster trust and mutual understanding among diverse professionals, thereby strengthening the capacity to support empowered, safe risk-taking.

Positive risk-taking also intersects with societal attitudes and stigma, particularly regarding disabled people, older adults, and those with mental health conditions. Historically, these groups have often been subject to overprotection, resulting in diminished independence and exclusion from decision-making. Challenging entrenched attitudes necessitates education and cultural change within care organisations, emphasising that independence and dignity are rights, not privileges, and that risk-taking is fundamental to living a fulfilling life. Promoting this culture shift involves leadership that champions innovation, encourages reflective practice, and supports staff to challenge the status quo. Celebrating successes and learning from challenges in positive risk-taking can foster optimism and resilience, driving ongoing improvements in care quality.

Critically, positive risk-taking does not mean ignoring risk but revaluing it as a necessary and beneficial element of life. It encourages creativity and flexibility in care planning, tailoring support to the unique needs and aspirations of everyone, rather than enforcing uniform safety policies that may inadvertently cause harm by limiting choice. It requires professionals to cultivate qualities such as empathy, intuition, cultural competence, and advocacy skills, enabling them to navigate complex human factors with confidence and sensitivity.

In everyday practice, supporting positive risk-taking might involve a care worker assisting a person with dementia in gardening independently, despite potential minor hazards, with measures in place for quick assistance if needed. Or it could mean enabling a young adult with physical disabilities to plan and undertake travel, recognising the empowering impact despite inherent risks. These examples highlight the essence of positive risk-taking: it is not about eliminating risk but about managing uncertainty to enable meaningful participation and fulfilment.

In conclusion, positive risk-taking embodies a compassionate, ethical commitment to supporting the rights and dignity of all service users by fostering empowerment, independence, and informed choice. It maintains a delicate balance between enabling freedom and ensuring protection through robust safeguarding practices and collaborative working. By embracing this approach, health and social care professionals contribute to a culture that values human potential, respects individuality, and advances the quality and humanity of care. This transformative perspective encourages all stakeholders to view risk not as an enemy to be avoided but as an element of life to be understood, managed, and sometimes embraced for the greater good.

Safeguarding and Risk

In the intricate landscape of health and social care, safeguarding is a paramount concern that is deeply intertwined with the principles of risk assessment and risk management. Safeguarding is the collective effort to protect the health, well-being, and human rights of individuals, enabling them to live free from abuse, harm, and neglect. Yet, it is a delicate balance to maintain one where the imperative to protect does not stifle the autonomy, independence, and dignity of those receiving care. This balance requires a profound understanding of the nuances of positive risk-taking alongside the readiness to recognise and respond to abuse in all its manifestations. Supporting independencc through positive risk-taking acknowledges that risk is an inherent part of everyday life and that attempting to eliminate all risk undermines the very essence of person-centred care. Every individual has the right to make decisions about their own lives, including accepting the risks that might accompany those choices. Health and social care professionals, therefore, are challenged to facilitate environments where service users can exercise autonomy safely, encouraging empowerment while vigilantly safeguarding against harm.

Recognising abuse and neglect is foundational to effective safeguarding and risk management. Abuse can take many forms, ranging from physical, emotional, sexual, and financial abuse to neglect, discriminatory practices, or institutional failings. The true complexity lies in the fact that abuse often occurs in contexts where trust and care should flourish. It may emerge subtly, hidden beneath layers of fear, dependency, or misinformation, thus demanding a heightened sensitivity from care providers. Recognising signs of abuse is not merely about noticing physical injuries or verbal disclosures; it also involves interpreting behavioural changes, emotional withdrawal, unexplained financial discrepancies, or deteriorations in personal hygiene and living conditions. These indicators often necessitate a holistic understanding of the individual's history, circumstances, and baseline well-being, underscoring the critical importance of building strong, trusting relationships between care providers and service users. Professionals must remain vigilant not only for evident signs but also for covert cues that suggest underlying safeguarding concerns.

Effective management of safeguarding risks requires a proactive, dynamic approach that goes beyond reactive responses. This begins with cultivating a culture of awareness and openness within care settings, where staff feel confident questioning, reporting, and discussing concerns without fear of reprisal. Risk assessments focused on safeguarding explore both internal and external factors that may predispose an individual to harm, combining this with strategies to mitigate those risks while upholding the person's rights and choices. Crucially, safeguarding risk management demands an understanding of the intersectionality of vulnerabilities wherein age, disability, mental health status, dependency, ethnicity, and socioeconomic factors converge to compound the risk. The framework for safeguarding must thus be flexible, person-centred, and attuned to the context-specific realities of each case. By embedding safeguarding considerations into routine risk assessment processes, care providers avoid compartmentalising safety concerns and instead foster a holistic approach in which every aspect of care delivery is scrutinised through a safeguarding lens.

Central to the safeguarding ethos in health and social care is the principle of multi-agency working, reflecting the recognition that no single organisation or professional has the full remit or capacity to address safeguarding issues effectively on their own. Collaborative partnerships are essential, uniting health professionals, social workers, law enforcement, regulatory bodies, advocacy groups, and even community organisations to form a comprehensive safety net for vulnerable individuals. Effective multi-agency working is predicated on clear communication channels, shared information protocols, and mutual respect for differing professional perspectives, roles, and responsibilities. A coordinated response ensures that risk assessments and safeguarding plans are thorough, timely, and reflective of a collective understanding of needs, risks, and protective factors. The benefits of such collaboration extend beyond immediate risk management; they contribute to building resilience within individuals and communities, promoting preventive strategies, and enhancing the quality and continuity of care.

Challenges to safeguarding and risk management often arise from systemic barriers such as conflicting priorities, bureaucratic complexities, resource constraints, and occasional inter-agency mistrust or territorialism. Overcoming these challenges requires sustained leadership commitment, continuous workforce training, and embedded accountability mechanisms. Empowering frontline workers with relevant knowledge of safeguarding legislation and best practices, and the skills to engage in sensitive conversations, is vital. Furthermore, organisations must cultivate environments that encourage and protect whistleblowing, ensuring that safeguarding concerns can surface without fear of retaliation or stigma. This cultural foundation supports staff in making difficult but necessary decisions about protective interventions, even when they involve complex ethical dilemmas or potential resistance from service users or their families.

The legislative framework in the UK provides a robust foundation for safeguarding within risk assessment, offering guidance and statutory duties that shape professional practice. Laws such as the Care Act 2014, the Children Act 1989 and 2004, the Safeguarding Vulnerable Groups Act 2006, and the Mental Capacity Act 2005 collectively establish the legal parameters within which risk must be assessed and managed. These statutes emphasise the importance of empowerment, prevention, proportionality, protection, partnership, and accountability, often referred to as the six principles of safeguarding. They mandate that safeguarding is not an afterthought but an integral part of care planning and delivery. Professionals are required to act in ways that promote well-being and independence while intervening decisively where there is a risk of significant harm. This legal foundation reinforces the moral imperative that safeguarding is everybody's responsibility in health and social care.

An often-overlooked dimension of safeguarding and risk is the need for detailed, accurate, and timely documentation and reporting. Comprehensive records ensure that safeguarding concerns are traceable, decisions about risk management are transparent, and there is continuity of communication among multi-agency partners. Documentation must be factual, objective, and free from personal bias, capturing the who, what, when, where, and how of incidents or observations that raise concerns. These records become critical evidence should investigations or legal proceedings ensue, underscoring the ethical obligation professionals carry to be meticulous and truthful. Moreover, reporting mechanisms must be accessible and widely understood by all staff, including clear pathways for escalation if immediate risks are identified. Training on recognising abuse, alongside guidance on confidentiality and information sharing, equips practitioners to navigate the complexities of safeguarding communications sensitively and lawfully.

Integral to safeguarding is appreciating the concept of positive risk-taking, which challenges traditional risk-averse attitudes in care. Rather than viewing risk solely as a threat to be eliminated, positive risk-taking recognises that some degree of risk is inherent in growth, autonomy, and quality of life. Care providers must therefore balance the potential harms against the benefits of supporting individuals in pursuing their goals, making choices, and engaging with their communities. This approach calls for nuanced risk assessments that explore scenarios creatively and collaboratively, involving service users, families, and relevant professionals in shared decision-making. It demands transparent discussions that honestly acknowledge risks while respecting an individual's right to take those risks knowingly. When done correctly, positive risk-taking can significantly enhance self-esteem, social inclusion, and overall well-being, transforming safeguarding from merely protection to a platform for empowerment.

In practice, safeguarding and risk assessment might involve considering a wide range of factors, such as the risks associated with a person's living arrangements, their mental and physical health, social networks, or activities they wish to undertake. For example, a service user with cognitive impairment may express a desire to undertake independent shopping trips. While this entails certain risks of forgetting items or encountering hazards, a blanket refusal could erode autonomy and confidence. Instead, a supporting risk assessment might identify practical controls, such as proper route planning, use of a mobile phone, or check-in systems, thereby managing risk without wholly curtailing independence. This illustrates how safeguarding is deeply connected to respect for individuality and tailored interventions.

The role of training and education in safeguarding against risks cannot be overstated. Staff at all levels benefit from continuous professional development that enhances their understanding of recognising abuse, implementing risk assessments, and fostering multi-agency collaboration. Scenario-based learning, reflective practice, and engagement with service users' experiences contribute to more empathetic, informed, and confident practitioners. As safeguarding landscapes evolve with emerging issues such as digital abuse or modern slavery, ongoing learning ensures that health and social care professionals remain equipped to address new challenges proactively.

Ultimately, safeguarding within risk assessment is a dynamic process requiring vigilance, compassion, and teamwork. It is about creating safe spaces where individuals can live with dignity, make their own choices with support, and be shielded from harm. By recognising abuse, managing safeguarding risks through comprehensive and individualised assessments, and embracing multi-agency collaboration, health and social care professionals forge the path towards safer, more inclusive care environments. This complex interplay between protection and empowerment defines the essence of safeguarding in modern practice, a commitment that embraces risk without succumbing to fear, enabling both safety and dignity to thrive together.

Building a Risk-Aware Culture

Creating and sustaining a risk-aware culture within health and social care settings is both an art and a science, demanding a multifaceted approach that intertwines knowledge, empathy, communication, and accountability. At its core, fostering such a culture begins with the recognition that risk in care environments is inevitable, but it need not be paralysing. Instead, when managed thoughtfully, risk-taking becomes a vehicle for empowerment, dignity, and enhanced quality of life for service users. Cultivating a risk-aware culture requires an environment where safety is prioritised without compromising the independence and autonomy of those receiving care. It calls for organisational commitment at all levels, from frontline practitioners to senior leadership, to embed continuous learning as a daily practice and not merely a procedural obligation.

Central to this is the delicate balance between safeguarding individuals and supporting positive risk-taking. Health and social care professionals must shift away from overly restrictive practices that may inadvertently diminish a person's sense of self and ability to make choices. Instead, by embracing calculated risks, professionals can encourage individuals to engage in activities that promote growth, learning, and well-being, recognising that absolute safety, while a worthy goal, is not always synonymous with quality care. This requires moving beyond traditional risk-averse mindsets and fostering an environment in which informed decisions are made collaboratively with service users, respecting their values and preferences. Professionals must work alongside individuals to understand which risks they are willing to accept and ensure that mitigation measures are in place to manage potential negative outcomes without infringing on autonomy.

Integral to nurturing a risk-aware culture is the proactive recognition and response to abuse and neglect. Raising awareness about the subtle signs of maltreatment ensures that care teams remain vigilant and prepared to intervene swiftly and effectively. This vigilance cannot reside solely with designated safeguarding leads but must permeate the entire workforce, cultivating a shared-responsibility ethos. Building this collective awareness involves comprehensive training that is routinely refreshed to reflect evolving threats and the complex realities of modern care environments. Furthermore, open channels of communication, where concerns can be voiced without fear of retribution, are vital to an organisation's safeguarding framework. When professionals feel supported to report suspicions or incidents, it creates a safer environment for all, enhancing trust within the team and among service users.

Managing safeguarding risks effectively demands an emphasis on transparency and ethical practice. This means not only recognising and responding to risk but also documenting actions meticulously to establish accountability and facilitate ongoing monitoring. High-quality record-keeping supports multi-agency collaboration, enabling external partners such as health services, law enforcement, and regulatory bodies to provide cohesive responses to safeguarding concerns. A risk-aware culture appreciates that safeguarding is dynamic; it unfolds over time and requires ongoing assessment and adjustment. It is not a static checklist but a living set of practices that evolve alongside the needs and contexts of those receiving care.

In this vein, inter-agency collaboration stands as a cornerstone of safety and quality in health and social care. Ensuring that information flows smoothly across professional boundaries demands mutual respect, shared objectives, and clarity of roles. Risk-aware organisations actively cultivate partnerships and trust with external agencies, recognising that safeguarding and risk management transcend singular domains. Regular multidisciplinary meetings, joint training sessions, and shared protocols help unify efforts and mitigate gaps or overlaps that might otherwise jeopardise service users' well-being. This collective approach ensures a holistic understanding of risk factors, facilitates comprehensive assessments, and promotes coordinated interventions that are responsive to the complexities of individuals' lives.

Embedding continuous learning within the organisation fuels a vibrant safety culture, where reflection on practice, openness to feedback, and willingness to adapt are paramount. Encouraging professionals to critically appraise incidents and near-misses without assigning blame fosters an environment where mistakes become catalysts for growth rather than sources of shame or fear.

Such learning mechanisms might include debriefings, development-focused supervision, and investment in professional education to keep risk management skills current and contextually relevant. Importantly, learning is not confined to internal personnel but extends to service users and their families. Engaging them as partners in understanding risks and protective factors deepens trust and enriches the risk assessment process with real-world insights.

Leadership plays an indispensable role in promulgating a risk-aware culture by modelling transparency, accountability, and empathy. Leaders who openly discuss risks and promote dialogue about challenges dismantle barriers that inhibit honest communication. Their commitment to safety is evident in the allocation of appropriate resources, the establishment of clear policies that support positive risk-taking, and the celebration of success stories in which risk management has enhanced service user outcomes. Moreover, leaders who prioritise well-being encourage staff to maintain resilience and guard against burnout, recognising that a fatigued workforce is less effective in identifying and managing risks.

The workforce itself is pivotal in cementing a risk-aware culture; as such, recruitment and retention strategies should focus on securing individuals who are not only skilled but also aligned with the organisation's values. Continuous professional development tailored to emerging risks, such as those related to digital technologies or social isolation, equips staff with contemporary tools and perspectives. Embedding reflective practice sessions where teams explore hypothetical risk scenarios allows them to rehearse responses and develop shared understandings. In doing so, ambiguity diminishes, and confidence flourishes, enabling care providers to act decisively and compassionately when confronted with real-world challenges.

Equally important is the role of communication in fostering a culture where risk is openly discussed without stigma or denial. Establishing forums for dialogue that include all stakeholders, care providers, service users, families, managers, and regulators creates a tapestry of voices that inform risk recognition and response. Such communication should be candid yet compassionate, acknowledging fears and concerns while collaboratively seeking solutions. When conversations about risk become routine and normalised rather than exceptional and fraught, the entire care environment benefits from increased transparency and mutual respect.

The physical environment also reflects and reinforces the cultural commitment to risk awareness. Designing care spaces that anticipate potential hazards and incorporate safety features that allow flexibility and autonomy signals an organisational dedication to balancing safety with independence. Accessibility and adaptability in environmental design empower individuals to engage with their surroundings confidently while reducing unnecessary restrictions. Moreover, organisational policies must embody this ethos by avoiding inflexible rules that stifle positive risk-taking and instead emphasise tailored approaches that respond to individuals' changing needs and capabilities.

In building a risk-aware culture, technology and data management systems emerge as valuable allies. Implementing digital tools that track incidents, flag emerging risks, and facilitate real-time communication between care teams can enhance responsiveness and precision in risk management. However, these systems must be implemented thoughtfully, ensuring that staff are comprehensively trained and that service users' privacy and dignity are safeguarded. Technology should augment, not replace, the human relationships central to effective risk assessment and care.

Sustaining a risk-aware culture is an ongoing journey rather than a destination. Regular audits, reviews, and quality improvement initiatives provide essential feedback loops, enabling organisations to identify patterns, anticipate challenges, and recalibrate strategies. Importantly, this responsiveness nurtures a sense of organisational agility, a readiness to adapt risk management practices considering evolving evidence, legislative changes, and societal expectations. A culture that embraces change as a pathway to improvement is better poised to protect all stakeholders while delivering care that is both safe and enriching.

Ultimately, building a risk-aware culture within health and social care requires an unwavering commitment to seeing risk not as a threat to be avoided at all costs but as an intrinsic part of life that, when approached with knowledge, respect, and courage, can support independence, dignity, and well-being. It is a culture that honours the complex humanity of both care providers and recipients, promotes multi-agency collaboration, champions safeguarding, and cultivates continuous learning. By embedding these principles into everyday practice and organisational ethos, care settings can transcend reactive risk management and move towards a proactive, inclusive, and dynamic environment where safety and empowerment coexist harmoniously.

Balancing Safety And Choice In Health And Social Care

In health and social care practice, one of the most complex and sensitive responsibilities is balancing safety with individual choice. Every day, practitioners are required to make decisions that protect individuals from harm while also respecting their rights, preferences, and independence. From my experience in the sector, I have noticed that this balance is not always easy to achieve. There are situations where prioritising safety may appear to conflict with a person's right to make their own decisions, and equally, promoting independence may introduce a level of risk.

The concept of balancing safety and choice is rooted in the principle of person-centred care. It recognises that individuals are not passive recipients of care but active participants in decisions about their lives. This approach aligns with the standards set by the Care Quality Commission (CQC), which emphasises dignity, respect, and individual autonomy. It also reflects the legal framework of the Mental Capacity Act 2005, which supports individuals in making their own decisions wherever possible, even when those decisions involve risk.

From what I have observed in practice, achieving this balance requires professional judgement, effective communication, and a clear understanding of both ethical and legal responsibilities. It is not about eliminating risk altogether, but about enabling individuals to live meaningful lives while minimising potential harm.

Understanding the Concept of Risk Enablement

Risk enablement is a key concept in balancing safety and choice. It involves supporting individuals in taking informed risks in ways that promote their independence and quality of life. Rather than adopting a risk-averse approach, practitioners work collaboratively with individuals to identify potential risks and develop strategies to manage them safely.

In my experience, risk enablement shifts the focus from "What could go wrong?" to "How can we support this safely?" For example, an older person may wish to continue cooking independently despite a risk of burns or fire. Instead of preventing them from cooking altogether, a risk-enabled approach would involve assessing risks and implementing measures such as supervision, safer equipment, or smoke alarms.

This approach not only enhances independence but also supports emotional well-being. I have noticed that when individuals feel in control of their lives, they are more confident, engaged, and satisfied with their care.

The Importance of Choice in Health and Social Care

Choice is fundamental to human dignity and autonomy. In health and social care, it encompasses decisions about daily routines, personal preferences, treatment options, and lifestyle choices. Respecting choice is essential for delivering person-centred care.

From my perspective, denying individuals the opportunity to make choices can lead to frustration, a loss of identity, and a reduced quality of life. For example, restricting a person's choice of clothing, food, or daily activities may seem minor, but over time, it can significantly impact their sense of self.

However, choice must be balanced with responsibility. Practitioners have a duty of care to protect individuals from harm, particularly when they are vulnerable. This creates a tension between promoting autonomy and ensuring safety.

Duty of Care and Professional Responsibility

Duty of care is a legal and ethical obligation to act in the best interests of individuals and to prevent foreseeable harm. In practice, this means that professionals must take reasonable steps to ensure safety while respecting individual rights.

I have found that the duty of care is often misunderstood as a requirement to eliminate all risks. It involves making informed decisions that balance risk and benefit. For example, allowing an individual to go out independently may involve some risk, but restricting their freedom entirely could be more harmful to their well-being.

Professionals must also be able to justify their decisions. This requires clear documentation, evidence-based practice, and adherence to organisational policies and procedures.

The Role of the Mental Capacity Act 2005

The Mental Capacity Act 2005 provides a framework for making decisions on behalf of individuals who may lack capacity. It is underpinned by five key principles, including the presumption of capacity and the right to make unwise decisions.

From my experience, one of the most important aspects of the Act is recognising that individuals have the right to take risks. Just because a decision appears unwise does not mean that the person lacks capacity.

When individuals lack capacity, decisions must be made in their best interests, considering their wishes, feelings, and values. This ensures that their rights and preferences are still respected.

Challenges in Balancing Safety and Choice

Balancing safety and choice presents several challenges in practice. One of the main challenges I have observed is the fear of blame or liability. Staff may adopt a risk-averse approach to avoid potential consequences, thereby limiting individuals' independence.

Another challenge is a lack of training or confidence. Without a clear understanding of risk assessment and legal frameworks, practitioners may struggle to make informed decisions.

Communication barriers can also create difficulties. If individuals are unable to express their preferences clearly, it becomes more challenging to support their choices.

Additionally, organisational pressures such as staff shortages and time constraints can impact the ability to carry out thorough risk assessments and provide personalised care.

Practical Approaches to Balancing Safety and Choice

From my experience, several strategies can support effective balancing of safety and choice in practice.

Firstly, person-centred risk assessments are essential. These assessments should involve the individual, their family, and relevant professionals. They should consider both risks and benefits and be regularly reviewed.

Secondly, effective communication is key. Practitioners must listen to individuals, understand their preferences, and provide clear information about risks and options.

Thirdly, training and support for staff are crucial. This includes understanding legal frameworks, developing risk assessment skills, and building confidence in decision-making.

Fourthly, organisations should promote a positive risk-taking culture. This involves supporting staff to make balanced decisions and recognising that some level of risk is acceptable.

Examples from Practice

In my role, I have encountered situations where balancing safety and choice required careful consideration. For instance, I worked with an individual who insisted on going out alone despite a history of falls. Rather than restricting their movement, we carried out a risk assessment, provided a walking aid, and arranged regular check-ins. This allowed the individual to maintain independence while reducing risk.

In another case, a service user with diabetes wanted to make their own dietary choices, including foods that could affect their condition. Instead of imposing restrictions, we provided education and support, enabling them to make informed decisions.

These examples highlight the importance of collaboration, communication, and flexibility in managing risk.

Ethical Considerations

Balancing safety and choice also involves ethical considerations. Principles such as autonomy, beneficence, non-maleficence, and justice must be considered.

Autonomy refers to respecting individuals' right to make their own decisions. Beneficence involves acting in their best interests, while non-maleficence focuses on avoiding harm. Justice ensures fairness and equality in care.

From my perspective, ethical practice requires a careful balance of these principles. It is not always possible to achieve a perfect solution, but decisions should be made transparently and with the individual's best interests in mind.

The Role of Leadership and Organisational Culture

Leadership plays a crucial role in promoting a balanced approach to safety and choice. Leaders must create an environment in which staff feel supported in making decisions and learning from experience.

In my experience, organisations with a strong culture of openness and learning are better able to manage risk effectively. This includes encouraging reporting of incidents, providing feedback, and continuously improving practice.

Policies and procedures should also support risk enablement rather than discourage it.

Conclusion

Balancing safety and choice in health and social care is a complex but essential aspect of practice. It requires a person-centred approach, informed decision-making, and a commitment to both safety and independence.

From what I have observed, the most effective approach is one that recognises the value of positive risk-taking and supports individuals to live meaningful lives. By working collaboratively, applying legal and ethical principles, and fostering a supportive organisational culture, practitioners can achieve a balance that protects individuals while respecting their rights.

Ultimately, making a difference in health and social care is not just about preventing harm, but about enabling people to live with dignity, choice, and purpose.

Legal Case Studies and Compliance

Landmark Legal Cases

The landscape of health and social care is continually shaped and refined by landmark legal cases that have highlighted both the profound responsibilities of care providers and the serious consequences of inadequate risk management. These cases not only underscore the importance of adherence to legal frameworks but also serve as critical learning tools, guiding professionals in making safer, more informed decisions. Examining these real-life instances allows an in-depth understanding of how failures in risk assessment and control have led to significant harm, legal liabilities, and reforms that resonate powerfully in daily practice.

One of the most influential cases in the history of health and social care risk management is the tragic story of "Donoghue v. Stevenson" (1932), which, though not directly a healthcare case, established the fundamental principle of duty of care that still governs modern practices. The case involved a consumer, Mrs. Donoghue, who became ill after drinking a ginger beer containing a decomposed snail. The court's ruling that manufacturers owe a duty of care to consumers laid the conceptual foundation for negligence claims in health and social care. It reminds care providers that their responsibilities extend beyond contractual obligations to a moral and legal duty to prevent harm to service users, setting a precedent that permeates risk assessment today.

Moving on to more contemporary and directly relevant cases, "R v. Occupational Health and Safety Executive, ex parte Huddersfield" (1993) highlights the real-world consequences of employers failing to uphold statutory health and safety standards. In this case, the employer's neglect in ensuring safe equipment and proper training led to a worker suffering serious injury. The legal verdict enforced the principle that care organisations must embed rigorous risk management processes as an integral part of their operational fabric, not merely as bureaucratic formalities. This case underscores that risk assessments are not optional but legally enforceable duties that require rigorous documentation and the proactive implementation of control measures.

In the realm of social care, the "Winterwerp case" (1979), a decision from the European Court of Human Rights, holds significant implications. It emphasised that deprivation of liberty must be lawful and that any restriction imposed on a person, such as a vulnerable individual in a care setting, must be necessary, proportionate, and subject to procedural safeguards. This ruling enshrined respect for personal autonomy and human rights within care provision, reinforcing the delicate balance between safeguarding and positive risk-taking. For risk assessors, the takeaway is clear: restrictions or interventions must be justified not only by safety concerns but also by legal and ethical standards recognising the service user's dignity and freedom.

The "Bolam test", originating from the case "Bolam v. Friern Hospital Management Committee" (1957), profoundly influences professional standards in healthcare risk management. The test sets the benchmark for determining whether a professional has met the acceptable standard of care by comparing their actions to those of a responsible body of peers. In practical terms, it means that care providers must align risk assessments and associated interventions with recognised, established practices, ensuring their approaches are defensible against scrutiny. This case serves as a protective shield for practitioners who follow accepted protocols, while also underscoring the need for continuous professional development to keep abreast of evolving standards and guidance.

Another pivotal legal episode is the "Montgomery v. Lanarkshire Health Board" (2015) decision, which transformed the approach to consent and information sharing, critical components of risk management in healthcare. The Supreme Court ruled that patients must be informed of any material risks involved in proposed treatments and reasonable alternatives, emphasising the ethos of respect for patient autonomy. This case shifted the responsibility onto healthcare providers to ensure transparent communication, making risk discussion a collaborative process. The practical implication for risk assessors is profound: service users must be actively involved and provided with clear, accessible information to make informed decisions, reinforcing the philosophy of empowerment and dignity at the heart of modern care.

Failures to manage risks appropriately often lead to devastating consequences, as starkly illustrated by the "Mid Staffordshire NHS Foundation Trust Public Inquiry" (2013). This inquiry unearthed systemic failures in care provision that led to unnecessary deaths and suffering due to inadequate staffing, poor governance, and negligent risk management practices. The findings highlighted how complacency, lack of transparency, and failure to act on warning signs can culminate in catastrophic outcomes. For care managers and frontline staff, this case serves as a sobering reminder that risk assessments must be dynamic and acted upon promptly, with organisational cultures promoting vigilance, accountability, and continuous improvement to safeguard service users effectively.

The “Winterbourne View” scandal further exposed the consequences when health and social care services abdicate their responsibility to manage and mitigate risks. Investigations revealed horrendous abuse of people with learning disabilities at a private hospital, exposing gross failures in safeguarding, supervision, and risk management by both the provider and oversight bodies. Legally, this ignited a nationwide conversation about the necessity for robust monitoring, whistleblowing policies, and multi-agency collaboration to detect and prevent abuse. Risk assessment here extends beyond physical hazards to encompass safeguarding risks, demanding comprehensive, person-centred, and ethically grounded approaches.

Equally instructive is the “Negligence claim following the death of Baby P” (Peter Connelly), which highlighted catastrophic failures in safeguarding children by social workers and health professionals. Despite multiple risk indicators and reports of abuse, inadequate assessment and communication failures culminated in a tragic loss. The subsequent public and legal scrutiny emphasised the critical importance of timely and accurate risk assessment, effective inter-agency communication, and mandatory escalation processes. For practitioners, this case underscores that risk assessment is not a static tick-box exercise but an active, ongoing process requiring vigilance and decisive action to protect vulnerable individuals.

The legal repercussions of poor risk management are further emphasised in cases involving medication errors and infection-control breaches, such as the “Liverpool Care Pathway” controversy, which led to significant legal and ethical reviews. The pathway, intended to provide compassionate end-of-life care, became synonymous with poor implementation and lack of informed consent, resulting in harm and distress. The fallout highlighted the necessity of incorporating risk assessment into clinical decision-making, including thorough evaluation of procedures, communication, and patient involvement, thereby illustrating that risks extend beyond physical safety to include psychological and emotional well-being.

Moreover, the case of “Nursing and Midwifery Council v. Rolfe” (2010) provides a stark illustration of the consequences of professional misconduct linked to inadequate risk management. The nurse, found guilty of negligent care leading to patient harm, faced suspension and legal censure. This outcome reinforces the message that individuals bear personal responsibility within the broader risk management framework and that professional standards demand the diligent application of risk assessment principles in everyday practice, from infection control to safeguarding.

Internationally, cases such as "X v. Finland" (2012), in which the European Court found that the state failed to adequately protect a vulnerable adult, extend the understanding of risk management failures as human rights violations. These legal rulings expand the sphere of risk assessment to encompass states' obligations and highlight the ethical imperative of care providers to adhere not only to national laws but also to international standards that uphold dignity and protection.

The synthesis of these landmark legal cases offers a compelling collective narrative on the evolution of risk management in health and social care. They illustrate that risk management failures may stem from varied sources: inadequate training, poor communication, insufficient documentation, cultural complacency, or broader systemic issues. Equally, they demonstrate that courts and regulatory bodies increasingly adopt a holistic view, recognising the interdependence of physical safety, safeguarding, legal compliance, and respect for autonomy. Consequently, risk assessments today cannot be simplistic but must be comprehensive, iterative, and person-centred, with active involvement from all stakeholders.

Practically, these cases provide clear guidance for health and social care professionals. They highlight the absolute necessity for thorough and regular risk assessments, well-documented and accessible records, and robust reporting mechanisms that escalate concerns swiftly and transparently. They demand that care providers foster a culture where positive risk-taking is balanced with safeguarding, autonomy is respected without compromising safety, and continuous professional development reinforces current best practices. Managers must ensure organisational compliance through training, supervision, and effective communication pathways, while regulatory agents must maintain vigilant oversight, leveraging lessons from past failures to inform future policy refinements.

In conclusion, landmark legal cases serve as critical mirrors reflecting the challenges and imperatives of risk management in health and social care. They chart the trajectory from foundational legal principles through the complexities of modern care environments, highlighting the profound ethical and legal responsibilities borne by providers. Their lessons resonate beyond courtrooms and into daily practice, urging all professionals to engage earnestly with risk assessment as a dynamic, essential function embedded in the fabric of care, one that protects service users, empowers practitioners, and sustains public trust. Embracing these lessons transforms risk assessment from a legal obligation into a proactive commitment to delivering safe, dignified, and high-quality care.

Ensuring Compliance

In the complex and highly regulated landscape of health and social care, ensuring compliance stands as both a critical obligation and a formidable challenge. At its core, compliance means adhering to a broad array of legislative, regulatory, and professional standards designed to safeguard the welfare of service users and protect care providers from preventable harm and liability. Meeting these standards is not merely about avoiding penalties or legal repercussions; it is fundamentally tied to delivering safe, dignified, and high-quality care. To grasp the full implication of compliance, one must appreciate that it is an ongoing, dynamic process, an intricate tapestry of policies, procedures, cultural attitudes, training, monitoring, and continual revision rather than a static checklist to be ticked off periodically.

The journey towards robust compliance begins with a clear understanding of the legal frameworks governing health and social care practice in the United Kingdom. Groundbreaking legislation such as the Health and Safety at Work Act 1974 lays down the foundation, establishing employers' and employees' responsibilities to protect health, safety, and welfare at work. Complemented by the Care Quality Commission (CQC) regulations and standards, these laws set explicit benchmarks for quality and safety tailored to service users' needs and contextual risks. However, it is the interplay between statute, guidance, and the ethical frameworks underpinning professional codes of conduct that shapes the practical demands placed on care organisations. Consequently, compliance is woven into every facet of operational management from risk assessment and training to communication and incident reporting. Without profound organisational commitment and clear leadership from managers, maintaining a culture that values and enforces compliance risks becoming a mere formality, prone to shortcuts and complacency.

Lessons learned from real legal cases vividly underscore the consequences of failing to meet risk management obligations. These cases reveal how neglecting compliance can translate into tragic outcomes for vulnerable service users and dire consequences for care providers, including criminal prosecution, civil lawsuits, and reputational damage. One poignant example is the case involving a care home where a lack of properly conducted risk assessments and inadequate staff training led to a resident's fatal injuries. The subsequent investigation uncovered systemic failures, including undocumented hazards and a culture that discouraged raising concerns. The court's judgment emphasised that compliance is about embedding safety in the very fabric of care, not simply reacting to incidents after they occur. This case and others reinforce the necessity for meticulous documentation and a proactive approach to identifying and mitigating risks. They also highlight the central role of whistleblowing policies in protecting service users and promoting transparency, where staff feel empowered and supported to report unsafe practices without fear of detriment.

To navigate the myriad complexities, organisations deploy diverse strategies and tools to maintain compliance. Integral to this is the development and implementation of thorough, accessible, and regularly updated policies and procedures that reflect current laws and best practices. These documents must be living instruments, shaped not only by legal requirements but also by the insights gained from audits, inspections, and service user feedback. For instance, the introduction of electronic risk management systems has transformed monitoring activities, with digital platforms enabling real-time data collection, automated review alerts, and centralised records accessible to multidisciplinary teams. Such technological integration enhances transparency and accountability while reducing human error and administrative burden. Equally important is tailoring these policies to specific care settings and populations, recognising that what applies in a residential care home differs from the nuances of community-based or mental health services. This contextual adaptation ensures relevance and effectiveness rather than superficial compliance.

A pivotal element of ensuring compliance is fostering a workforce culture deeply committed to safety and accountability. Managers and senior leaders bear a significant responsibility to instil this ethos by prioritising training that goes beyond one-off sessions towards continuous professional development embedded in daily practice. Training should encompass not only the procedural aspects of risk assessments and reporting but also the cultivation of critical thinking skills, ethical awareness, and an understanding of the broader societal impact of their roles. Moreover, compliance is enhanced when staff at all levels recognise the importance of collaboration and open communication, encouraged through regular team meetings, reflective practice, and multi-agency partnerships. Organisations that promote a "just culture" – where errors are openly discussed and used as learning opportunities rather than occasions for punitive measures – tend to see increased incident reporting and safer care. This cultural approach aligns with the principles of continuous improvement, ensuring that compliance evolves in step with emerging challenges and changing legislation.

Internal and external audit mechanisms serve as essential tools for verifying compliance and identifying areas for improvement. Routine internal audits, including detailed reviews of risk assessment documentation, incident logs, and policy adherence, provide managers with insight into practice gaps and training needs. These processes should be systematic, thorough, and interpreted in the context of the organisation's risk profile and service user population. Alongside these, external audits and inspections conducted by agencies such as the CQC provide authoritative assessments of compliance and can influence publicly available regulatory ratings, affecting both reputation and funding streams. The inspection process encourages transparency and drives improvement, but it can also be a source of stress if organisations are poorly prepared or fail to engage meaningfully with reviewers. To mitigate this, cultivating a culture of readiness, not preparedness, solely for inspections, but readiness for everyday accountability, is crucial. That is, organisations should embed compliance in routine practice rather than treating audits as episodic events.

Beyond formal audits, the active analysis of incidents, near misses, and complaints provides a wealth of intelligence for refining compliance strategies. Incident investigations should adopt a systematic and impartial approach, focusing on identifying root causes rather than assigning blame, ensuring lessons learned translate into concrete action. For example, if a medication error is traced back to insufficient staff training or unclear protocols, immediate remediation coupled with enhanced supervision and revised procedures is necessary. Recording these actions transparently in quality assurance frameworks evidences a commitment to learning and public accountability. Importantly, this feedback loop must include service users and their families wherever possible, respecting their perspectives as essential components of comprehensive risk assessment and compliance review.

The legal environment itself is continually evolving, and organisations must be agile in responding to new regulations, statutory guidance, and judicial precedents. For instance, changes in safeguarding legislation, standards relating to mental capacity, or pandemic-related infection control measures demand rapid incorporation into operational policies and training. Staying current, therefore, hinges on proactive information gathering, often through networks such as professional associations, regulatory updates, and sector-specific forums. Some organisations appoint dedicated compliance officers or risk managers whose sole remit is to monitor these developments and coordinate organisational responses. This specialist role becomes critical in larger entities where complexity and rapid change could otherwise overwhelm generalist managers. However, in smaller care settings, shared responsibility and effective communication channels are equally vital. Creating mechanisms for staff to voice concerns promptly enables early identification of emerging compliance risks.

Technology also offers innovative avenues for supporting compliance beyond documentation and monitoring. E-learning platforms, for example, allow staff to access updated training materials flexibly, track progress, and demonstrate competency through assessments. Similarly, mobile applications with decision-support tools empower care workers in real time, guiding them through risk-assessment steps and prompting critical safety checks at the point of care. These digital innovations, when thoughtfully integrated, reduce reliance on memory, standardise procedures, and foster uniform practice standards across teams. Yet, technological adoption must be accompanied by robust data governance policies to ensure confidentiality and security, especially when handling sensitive personal or health information.

Leadership commitment is the linchpin that holds all these elements together into an effective compliance framework. Leaders in health and social care must visibly champion compliance initiatives, allocate adequate resources, and model behaviours that reinforce safety and ethical care. When compliance is perceived as a strategic organisational priority rather than a bureaucratic requirement, it permeates daily operations and influences decision-making. This leadership approach also facilitates the balancing of compliance with positive risk-taking, the delicate task of enabling service users' independence while managing potential hazards. Strong leadership promotes open dialogue about risks and encourages innovation in care planning that respects individual rights yet maintains protection.

In summary, ensuring compliance requires a multifaceted, proactive approach that integrates legal knowledge, organisational culture, staff competence, technological tools, and leadership engagement. The repercussions of lapses, underscored by real cases where failures had devastating effects, serve as sober reminders of the stakes involved. Yet, these experiences also guide the continuous refinement of strategies that turn legal obligations into practical safety nets, embedding risk management into the heart of care delivery. For health and social care providers, achieving compliance is more than a target; it is an evolving commitment to excellence, safeguarding, and respect for those they serve.

Consequences of non-compliance

Non-compliance in health and social care settings carries profound, often devastating consequences, extending far beyond immediate operational challenges to reverberate across legal, professional, and moral dimensions. At its core, failure to adhere rigorously to established risk assessment protocols and regulatory mandates jeopardises not only the health and well-being of service users but also the safety of care providers, organisations, and the broader community. Legal ramifications are among the most tangible and severe outcomes, with the potential to involve criminal prosecutions, civil litigation, monetary penalties, and formal sanctions such as license revocation or suspension. These repercussions serve as stark reminders that compliance is not merely a bureaucratic exercise but an essential element of ethical and effective care delivery.

Delving into the legal landscape reveals numerous illustrative cases that underscore the critical importance of maintaining stringent compliance with risk assessment frameworks. One landmark case involved a care home where systemic failure to properly assess and mitigate risks related to residents' mobility led to a serious injury and subsequent legal action exposing significant lapses in organisational accountability. The court found that inadequate staff training, poor documentation, and a lack of rigorous hazard identification collectively amounted to gross negligence. The resulting judgment not only imposed substantial damages on the care provider but also triggered closer regulatory scrutiny and demanded immediate remedial action. This case illuminated how omissions, often perceived as administrative oversights, could escalate into catastrophic events with both human and financial costs. The lesson drawn is unequivocal: consistent, documented risk assessment processes are foundational to preventing harm and guarding against legal vulnerabilities.

Similarly, the tragic inquiries into high-profile institutional failings have repeatedly highlighted the devastating consequences when risk management systems are neglected or superficially implemented. The public inquiries following certain hospital scandals exposed systemic failures to identify and address risks related to patient safety, inadequate infection control practices, and failure to safeguard vulnerable individuals. These inquiries revealed that despite existing policies, operational cultures lacked the commitment and oversight needed to translate risk assessment into actionable safety measures. Professional regulators consequently imposed disciplinary measures against individuals and organisations, including suspension of practice and mandatory retraining, emphasising that non-compliance is not tolerated at any level within the health and social care sector. Beyond legal penalties, these incidents damaged public trust, eroding confidence in care providers and exacerbating the distress experienced by affected service users and their families, thereby underscoring the far-reaching societal impact of non-compliance.

From a professional standpoint, the ramifications extend into the realm of individual accountability and career sustainability. Care staff and management bear personal responsibility for the implementation and oversight of risk assessments under regulatory expectations. Non-compliance can lead to investigations by professional bodies, which may result in cautions, reprimands, suspension, or even removal from professional registers and licensing bodies. Such outcomes not only carry immediate punitive effects but also have long-term career implications, restricting future employment opportunities and reputation within the sector. More subtly, instances of non-compliance can erode workplace morale, increase staff turnover, and undermine the collective commitment to quality care. The professional isolation and stigma associated with breaches of risk management standards serve as powerful deterrents, reinforcing the importance of vigilance, continuing education, and adherence to best practices.

Beyond individual and organisational consequences, there are broader ethical and societal considerations that compound the significance of compliance. Failure to properly assess and manage risks undermines the fundamental principle of care, the safeguarding of human dignity and well-being. When service users suffer due to ignored or poorly executed risk assessments, the damage to their trust, autonomy, and sense of security can be profound and enduring. Such outcomes contravene the ethical obligations enshrined in health and social care codes of conduct and can precipitate a breakdown in therapeutic relationships, further complicating care delivery and recovery. Societal costs also manifest through the increased burden on health systems, families, and communities as preventable injuries and neglect result in additional interventions, hospital admissions, and resource allocation challenges. Consequently, compliance is integral not only to legal adherence but to the ethical stewardship of care responsibilities.

Practical guidance on maintaining compliance is anchored in a proactive approach that embeds risk assessment as a continuous, dynamic process rather than a periodic administrative task. Effective compliance starts with comprehensive training tailored to different levels of responsibility, ensuring that all staff, from frontline care providers to senior management, understand the principles, legislative requirements, and organisational policies governing risk assessment. This education must be reinforced regularly, adapting to evolving legal standards, emerging risks, and lessons learned from incidents and near-misses. Monitoring and auditing systems play a vital role in detecting lapses early, offering opportunities for corrective action before issues escalate. Clear reporting mechanisms, including whistleblowing policies, encourage transparency and early identification of non-compliance without fear of retribution, thereby fostering a culture of accountability and openness.

Documentation practices represent another cornerstone in maintaining compliance. Detailed, accurate, and up-to-date records of risk assessments, incidents, and control measures demonstrate due diligence and provide essential evidence in the event of legal scrutiny. Integrated electronic systems facilitate real-time data capture and analysis, supporting risk prioritisation and resource allocation. Importantly, involving service users and their families in the risk assessment process through shared decision-making and transparent communication ensures that risk management is person-centred, respectful, and legally sound. Engagement enhances understanding and acceptance of necessary risk controls, reducing resistance and enhancing adherence to safety protocols.

Multi-agency collaboration further strengthens compliance frameworks by pooling expertise, resources, and oversight. Social workers, healthcare professionals, regulatory agents, and community organisations all contribute unique perspectives and capabilities to comprehensive risk management. Establishing clear lines of communication, shared responsibilities, and joint training initiatives promotes consistency and reduces fragmentation that can lead to oversights. Particularly in safeguarding scenarios, coordinated strategies are essential for timely intervention and prevention of harm. Regulatory bodies themselves provide guidance, support, and enforcement that underpin compliance efforts; active engagement with these agencies can help organisations anticipate regulatory changes and embed best practices.

Ultimately, embracing a positive risk culture that values ethical accountability, continuous improvement, and reflective practice is the most effective safeguard against the dire consequences of non-compliance. Leadership commitment is crucial: setting expectations, modelling compliance behaviours, and adequately resourcing necessary systems. This cultural foundation supports practitioners in balancing necessary risks with safety, encourages innovation in care practices, and legitimises honest reflection on mistakes and near misses as learning opportunities. In doing so, organisations not only avert legal and professional ramifications but also drive improvements in the quality of care and better outcomes for service users.

In summary, the consequences of non-compliance in risk assessment within health and social care are multifaceted and substantial. Legal repercussions, including prosecution and civil action, highlight the gravity of failing to meet statutory duties. Professional sanctions underscore the individual responsibility borne by care practitioners beyond organisational mandates. Ethical breaches erode the trust and dignity fundamental to effective care, with wider societal costs in terms of resources and community well-being. By learning from real-world failures and adopting robust training, documentation, reporting, and collaborative practices, care providers can build resilient compliance frameworks. These, underpinned by a supportive culture, serve not only to meet regulatory demands but to genuinely make a positive difference in the care and protection of vulnerable individuals. The stakes are high, but the pathway to safe, dignified, and legally sound care is clear and attainable through committed, collective action.

Technology in Risk Assessment

Digital Tools Overview

In the contemporary landscape of health and social care, digital tools have emerged as an indispensable ally in the quest to manage risks comprehensively and efficiently. The increasing complexity of care environments demands not only vigilance but also sophisticated methods for identifying, assessing, and controlling potential hazards while maintaining meticulous documentation. Technology here serves not merely as a convenience but as a vital piece of infrastructure that enhances accuracy, responsiveness, and collaboration among care providers, managers, and regulatory bodies. As such, digital tools encompass a broad spectrum of technologies ranging from specialised software platforms designed to streamline risk assessment processes to mobile applications that enhance real-time data capture and response. Additionally, an array of digital tracking methods, including wearable devices and sensor systems, empowers health and social care professionals to monitor conditions in real time, anticipate risks before they escalate, and implement precautionary measures with greater precision.

Central to this technological transformation is the proliferation of risk management software tailored explicitly for care settings. These platforms are designed to guide users through the intricate processes of hazard identification and risk evaluation while ensuring compliance with legal and organisational standards. They often feature integrated databases that securely store information about service users, specific risk factors, and past incidents, which can be cross-referenced. This capability enables practitioners to draw informed conclusions based on historical patterns and comparative analyses. Moreover, such software frequently incorporates automated or semi-automated risk-rating tools that utilise risk matrices or likelihood-versus-severity calculations to prioritise the urgency of different hazards. By automating parts of these calculations, the technology reduces human error and streamlines what can otherwise be a cumbersome cognitive task. Importantly, these systems can be configured to send alerts and reminders for the review and updating of risk assessments, thereby fostering a culture of continuous improvement and regulatory compliance.

Many of these platforms go beyond static documentation, embracing collaborative functionalities that facilitate communication across multi-disciplinary teams. In health and social care settings where various professionals interact, nurses, social workers, therapists, and managers, ensuring consistent, accessible, and up-to-date information is crucial. Cloud-based systems, in particular, enable simultaneous access to risk assessments, care plans, and incident reports, removing traditional silos and delays. This real-time accessibility not only enhances the quality of decision-making but also reinforces accountability by providing transparent records of who entered the data, when changes were made, and how risks were controlled. Furthermore, these tools often integrate with broader organisational or regulatory databases, aiding in the collection of mandatory compliance data and facilitating reporting to bodies such as the Care Quality Commission.

Complementing desktop and enterprise software, mobile applications have redefined the flexibility and immediacy with which risk assessments are conducted and updated. These applications are especially valuable in dynamic or community-based care environments where practitioners move between locations or encounter rapidly changing circumstances. Smartphone or tablet apps provide user-friendly interfaces to perform on-the-spot risk evaluations, capture images or voice notes to provide accurate context, and submit reports instantly via secure networks. By enabling dynamic risk assessment, these apps empower care providers to respond promptly to emerging hazards, ensuring safety measures evolve alongside real-world conditions. The incorporation of GPS features and geofencing within some apps further enhances compliance and safety monitoring, for example, by alerting managers if lone workers stray beyond designated safe areas or fail to check in as required.

Infection control, a paramount concern in health and social care, has also been bolstered by sophisticated digital tracking tools. Contact tracing applications and electronic symptom trackers, while widely recognised for their pandemic-related roles, have lasting relevance in preventing and managing infectious disease outbreaks in care facilities. These digital tools enable rapid identification of potential exposure chains, supporting timely isolation and intervention strategies. By integrating with electronic health records, these systems help maintain comprehensive, up-to-date profiles of service users' health status and vaccination histories, thereby informing individualised risk assessments that reflect current epidemiological realities.

Among the most cutting-edge technologies driving risk management are wearable devices and sensor-based systems that continuously monitor physiological and environmental parameters. These technologies provide proactive rather than reactive data, shifting the paradigm of risk assessment from episodic to continuous surveillance. Wearables such as smartwatches and biosensors can track vital signs, detect falls, monitor mobility, and even gauge emotional states through biometric indicators. This real-time physiological data, when transmitted securely to central monitoring hubs, enables rapid intervention in emergencies, reducing adverse outcomes. Similarly, environmental sensors detect smoke, gas leaks, temperature fluctuations, or movement anomalies within a facility, triggering automated alerts or activating prevention controls. These systems are particularly beneficial for vulnerable service users who may be cognitively impaired or unable to communicate hazards independently. By embedding digital vigilance into the care environment itself, these tools provide an additional protective layer that supports traditional risk assessment protocols.

The utility of digital tools extends to documentation and regulatory compliance, which are critical components of risk management frameworks. Traditional paper-based forms are susceptible to loss, damage, and inconsistencies, whereas electronic documentation ensures data integrity, searchability, and secure storage. Digital forms and reporting tools often incorporate mandatory fields and validation checks to minimise incomplete or inaccurate entries. This rigour is essential when documenting incidents, near misses, or safeguarding concerns, as precise records form the foundation for legal accountability and quality improvement. Advanced systems facilitate automatic generation of comprehensive reports tailored to specific regulatory requirements, thereby easing the administrative burden on care providers and enabling timely submission to oversight agencies. Moreover, electronic systems support audit trails that demonstrate compliance over time, enhancing organisational transparency and fostering regulatory trust.

Artificial intelligence (AI) and machine learning are beginning to influence risk management by offering predictive analytics capabilities that analyse large datasets to uncover patterns beyond human capacity. These technologies can process diverse inputs from incident logs to physiological monitoring to forecast potential risk escalations or identify latent hazards. For instance, AI-powered platforms could flag service users at heightened risk of falls or medication errors before these events occur, using historical data and real-time inputs. While their integration is still evolving in health and social care, these innovations herald a future where technology operates as a proactive partner in safeguarding and quality assurance, continuously refining risk controls and enhancing personalised care plans.

It is important to note, however, that the effective deployment of these digital tools requires thoughtful attention to usability, accessibility, and training. The care workforce varies widely in digital literacy, and technologies must be intuitive and responsive to the unique workflows and environments endemic to health and social care. User-friendly design that accommodates diverse abilities and integrates seamlessly with existing care routines ensures greater adoption and ultimately, better risk management outcomes. Equally vital is the assurance of data security and confidentiality. Handling sensitive personal and health information demands robust encryption, access controls, and compliance with data protection regulations such as the General Data Protection Regulation (GDPR). Trust in these systems hinges on safeguarding personal dignity and privacy, in parallel with the broader commitment to empowering service users amid risk-control efforts.

Collectively, the spectrum of digital tools from sophisticated risk management software and collaborative cloud platforms to mobile apps, wearable sensors, and AI-driven analytics has transformed how health and social care professionals approach risk. These technologies serve not only as enablers of more detailed and timely risk assessments but also as catalysts for stronger communication, enhanced service user involvement, and improved regulatory compliance. They facilitate a shift towards a more proactive, responsive, and person-centred risk management culture that can accommodate the complexities of modern care environments. As digital capabilities continue to expand, their integration into everyday practice promises to refine the balance between safeguarding and empowerment, ensuring that risks are managed not through rigidity but through smart, adaptive, and humane approaches that respect the dignity and independence of those receiving care.

Implementing Technology

Embracing technology in health and social care risk assessment is no longer a futuristic concept but a pressing necessity that can fundamentally transform how professionals approach safety, compliance, and wellbeing. Implementing digital tools requires more than simply purchasing software or devices; it demands a thoughtful, strategic integration into everyday practice, ensuring these innovations enhance, not hinder, the complex work environment. The journey toward successful technological adoption begins with a comprehensive understanding of the specific needs and challenges faced by the care setting, as this dictates which digital offerings will provide the most meaningful support. Whether a care provider is seeking to improve the accuracy of hazard identification, streamline assessment workflows, bolster control measures, or ensure airtight documentation, there exists a diverse landscape of technology solutions designed to meet these goals. Yet, for these benefits to materialise, the introduction of technology must be deliberate, person-centred, and inclusive of the entire workforce.

To kickstart the process of integrating technology into risk assessment, it is imperative to engage key stakeholders early on. Managers and frontline care staff should be involved in candid discussions about current pain points within risk identification and management. This collaborative dialogue helps to illuminate gaps in existing systems, offering insight into the types of digital interventions that would be most valuable. For instance, care providers struggling with inconsistent hazard reporting could explore mobile applications that allow immediate, on-the-spot documentation. Similarly, teams overwhelmed by mountains of paperwork might benefit from software that consolidates assessments and flags risks through automated alerts and risk matrix visualisations. By aligning technological goals with the lived realities of those conducting assessments and caring for service users, organisations lay a foundation for acceptance and ownership of new tools, an essential ingredient for sustainable implementation.

Once the needs assessment establishes the direction for technology adoption, selecting the appropriate tools requires a careful evaluation of functionality, user-friendliness, and interoperability with existing systems. In health and social care, digital risk assessment platforms often come equipped with modules for hazard identification checklists, automated risk scoring, control measure tracking, and real-time reporting dashboards. These features are designed not only to aid in comprehensive assessments but also to facilitate quicker responses to emerging risks. However, the complexity of such software can easily overwhelm users if the interface is cumbersome or if essential features require a high level of technical proficiency. Thus, priority should be given to solutions that balance robust capability with simplicity, ensuring that even practitioners with limited digital experience can navigate tools confidently. Moreover, compatibility with other platforms, such as electronic health records or incident management systems, is vital to avoid creating siloed information repositories that fragment care continuity and reporting accuracy.

With a selected digital tool, the focus naturally shifts to equipping the workforce through thorough, tailored training programs. Effective training transcends basic operational instructions, delving into how the technology integrates with existing workflows and enhances the quality of risk assessment. Care providers should be encouraged to appreciate how digital solutions help capture nuances often missed in manual recordkeeping, such as trend analyses over time or automatic flagging of escalating hazards. Training sessions designed to reflect the diversity of learner styles, combining live demonstrations, hands-on practice, video tutorials, and written guides, can significantly enhance engagement and retention. Importantly, training should address potential anxieties or resistance related to fears of job displacement or increased surveillance, reassuring staff that technological tools empower their judgement rather than replace it. Cultivating digital champions within teams, enthusiastic early adopters who can mentor peers and model positive attitudes toward technology, further smooths the transition and supports long-term proficiency.

Beyond initial training, ongoing support mechanisms are indispensable for cementing digital competence and fostering confidence. Establishing help desks or dedicated IT support lines focused on risk assessment technology provides immediate assistance when users encounter difficulties, preventing frustration and task abandonment. Regular refresher sessions and opportunities for feedback allow organisations to identify usability issues, adapt training materials, and highlight new features or updates. Additionally, embedding technology use into everyday supervision and appraisal discussions sends a powerful message that digital risk assessment is integral to quality care, encouraging continuous improvement in both technical skill and clinical judgement. Care managers can harness software-generated usage analytics to monitor how staff engage with digital tools, identify gaps in adoption, and tailor support accordingly, thereby creating a responsive learning environment that evolves alongside technological advancements.

On the practical side, implementing technology also involves reconfiguring workflows to accommodate digital processes without disrupting care delivery. For example, paper-based risk assessments traditionally occur at set intervals or post-incident, but with mobile applications and cloud-based platforms, assessments can become dynamic, real-time activities seamlessly integrated into daily routines. Devices such as tablets or smartphones enable care providers to document hazards and control measures on the spot, complete with photos, voice recordings, or GPS tagging to provide richer contextual information. This immediacy not only enhances accuracy but also allows rapid dissemination of risk information to all relevant parties, promoting timely intervention. It is crucial, however, to ensure that technological adoption does not add undue burden; thus, systems should be designed with flexible interfaces that allow quick entry, multiple languages or accessibility settings, and offline functionality for settings with limited internet connectivity.

Data security and confidentiality are paramount considerations in any digital transformation within health and social care, given the sensitive nature of risk assessment records. Implementing technology mandates robust cybersecurity protocols, including encrypted data transmission, secure login credentials, and strict user access controls to prevent unauthorised viewing or manipulation of records. Training must explicitly cover these data protection measures and the legal ramifications of breaches under frameworks such as the UK Data Protection Act and GDPR. Organisations should conduct regular audits to ensure compliance and adapt policies as new threats emerge. Furthermore, a culture of transparency regarding data use reassures staff and service users alike that technology operates within ethical boundaries that respect privacy and consent.

In tandem with security, technology offers unprecedented opportunities for collaboration within and beyond the care setting. Digital platforms can facilitate multi-agency risk assessment by providing shared access to key information among healthcare professionals, social workers, regulatory agents, and emergency responders, breaking down silos that traditionally hampered coordinated care efforts. Features such as live dashboards, integrated messaging, and centralised document repositories streamline communication, ensuring that everyone involved has timely visibility of risks and management plans. This interconnectivity not only improves the speed and efficacy of responses but also supports comprehensive safeguarding, as concerns can be escalated promptly via standardised digital protocols.

Despite the clear advantages, organisations must remain mindful of challenges intrinsic to technological change. Resistance rooted in fear of complexity or loss of personal interaction, limited staff digital literacy, initial financial costs, and the risk of overreliance on software algorithms to replace human judgment are common hurdles. These concerns underscore the importance of maintaining a balanced approach in which technology serves as an enabler rather than a replacement for professional expertise and compassionate care. Continuous dialogue, patient and service user involvement, and adaptability to feedback ensure that digital tools evolve in harmony with both practitioner capabilities and ethical standards.

Ultimately, adopting technology in risk assessment represents a meaningful stride toward enhancing safety, efficiency, and accountability within health and social care. From initial needs analysis and stakeholder engagement through careful tool selection, comprehensive training, workflow redesign, and robust support, each phase demands attention and commitment. When implemented thoughtfully, digital innovations empower care providers to identify hazards earlier, assess risks more accurately, implement controls effectively, and document processes transparently, thereby improving outcomes for service users. Embracing technology with a conscientious, people-centred ethos paves the way for a future where risk assessment is not just a regulatory obligation but a dynamic, integrated pillar of exceptional and compassionate care delivery.

Challenges and Solutions

In the dynamic and often unpredictable realm of health and social care, professionals continually confront a range of challenges when conducting risk assessments. These challenges stem not only from the inherent complexities of human needs and care environments but also from systemic, technological, and resource-related barriers. Understanding and addressing these obstacles requires a thoughtful blend of traditional approaches with innovative technological advancements designed to optimise the thoroughness and effectiveness of risk identification, assessment, control, and documentation. The integration of digital tools such as software platforms, mobile applications, and real-time tracking systems has the potential to revolutionise how professionals manage risk, promoting safer, more efficient, and more person-centred care.

One of the earliest and most persistent challenges in risk assessment involves the accurate and timely identification of potential hazards. In many traditional settings, this process relies heavily on manual observation, reporting, and subjective judgment, which can be inconsistent and vulnerable to human error or oversight. The busy nature of care environments, combined with staffing pressures and fluctuating service user needs, often means that risks may go unnoticed or unreported until they manifest in adverse outcomes. Moreover, communication gaps between care teams, managers, and external agencies may further hinder the swift recognition and response to emerging hazards. Addressing this challenge demands the deployment of technology that supports more systematic, real-time, and collaborative risk identification methods.

Software solutions have become increasingly sophisticated, offering dashboards and alert systems that aggregate data from multiple sources within the care setting. For instance, integrated platforms can pull information from electronic health records, incident reports, environmental sensors, and feedback forms, creating a comprehensive and dynamic snapshot of current risks. This holistic data integration allows care providers and managers to detect patterns and trends that might otherwise remain hidden, enabling proactive interventions. These platforms often include customisable risk assessment templates tailored to different care contexts and user needs, streamlining data entry and ensuring consistent documentation across teams. When combined with role-based access controls and audit trails, such software not only enhances data security and privacy compliance but also facilitates accountability and transparency.

Mobile applications further enhance risk management by enabling frontline staff to report concerns promptly, often via user-friendly devices such as smartphones and tablets. This immediacy reduces communication delays and empowers care workers to contribute actively to safety culture. Apps equipped with voice recognition and photographic capabilities allow for richer, more detailed reporting, capturing nuances that written notes may miss. Some applications incorporate checklists and guided prompts aligned with best-practice standards, helping users adhere to structured assessment processes even under time constraints or in high-pressure situations. Additionally, apps may include multilingual support or accessibility features, ensuring inclusivity and comprehension across diverse workforces.

Digital tracking methods also play a crucial role in continuous risk monitoring and control. Wearable devices, environmental sensors, and location-based technologies can collect objective data on factors such as movement patterns, physiological indicators, or room temperatures. For example, sensor systems installed in care homes can detect falls or unusual activity, prompting immediate alerts to care staff. When linked with risk management software, these inputs contribute to an evolving risk profile for each service user or care area. This real-time monitoring enables dynamic risk assessments that adapt to changing conditions, rather than relying solely on periodic manual reviews. The capacity for continuous assessment supports early intervention, reducing the likelihood of harm.

While the potential of technology in risk assessment is significant, its adoption is not without obstacles. Care settings often face limited financial resources, which restrict investment in new digital systems or the necessary infrastructure, like reliable internet connectivity and up-to-date hardware. Smaller organisations, or those operating in rural or deprived areas, may experience these disadvantages more acutely, thereby widening disparities in care safety standards. Resistance from staff who may be unfamiliar with, uncomfortable with, or sceptical of new technologies is another barrier, especially if implementation is perceived as adding to their workload or threatening their job security. Successful integration requires comprehensive training, ongoing support, and cultural change initiatives that promote technology as a tool for empowerment rather than surveillance. Engaging practitioners in the design or selection of systems can enhance ownership and usability.

Data security and confidentiality concerns are paramount, given the sensitive nature of health and social care information. Digital solutions must comply rigorously with UK data protection legislation, such as the General Data Protection Regulation (GDPR) and the Data Protection Act 2018. This necessitates robust encryption, secure access protocols, and clear policies outlining data collection, storage, sharing, and disposal. Any breach of confidentiality can have serious implications for service user trust, staff morale, and organisational reputation. Care organisations must balance the benefits of comprehensive digital data collection with stringent safeguards to maintain legal and ethical standards.

To overcome these challenges, organisations are increasingly adopting hybrid approaches that combine the strengths of technology with human judgment and flexibility. For example, digital tools may handle routine data capture and analysis, while frontline staff retain responsibility for nuanced interpretation and decision-making. This partnership ensures that technology enhances rather than replaces professional expertise. Moreover, automated reminders and alerts prompt timely review and updating of risk assessments, counteracting the tendency for paperwork to become outdated or neglected in busy settings. Integration of incident reporting systems with risk registers allows a seamless flow from event identification through to evaluation and learning, fostering a continuous improvement cycle.

Emerging technologies such as artificial intelligence (AI) and machine learning promise further advancements in risk assessment by enabling predictive analytics. These systems can analyse vast datasets to identify subtle correlations and forecast potential risks before they escalate. For instance, AI algorithms might detect early indicators of infection outbreaks within care facilities or flag increased fall risk based on changes in a resident's mobility data. Such predictive capacity shifts the paradigm from reactive to preventative care, aligning with broader healthcare goals of reducing harm and optimising resource use. Nonetheless, these technologies must be carefully validated and monitored to avoid biases or errors that could lead to inappropriate risk categorisation or over-reliance on automated outputs.

Collaboration across agencies and sectors is also facilitated by digital platforms designed to support multi-agency working. Secure portals allow information sharing while respecting confidentiality and consent parameters, ensuring that all relevant parties, from social workers and medical professionals to emergency responders and family members, have access to up-to-date risk information. This coordination enhances holistic understanding and management of risks that span organisational boundaries, such as safeguarding concerns or complex health conditions. It also prevents duplication of effort and streamlines communication channels, reducing frustration and delays.

In practical terms, organisations can optimise the use of technology in risk assessment by investing in comprehensive needs analyses before selecting software or tools, ensuring alignment with organisational goals, user workflows, and regulatory requirements. Pilot testing and phased rollouts allow iterative refinement and the opportunity to address unforeseen challenges. Regular feedback loops involving end users support continuous improvement and adaptation to evolving practice demands. Training programs that focus not only on technical operations but also on underlying risk management principles foster meaningful engagement and skill development.

Another vital solution is to embed risk assessment technology within broader quality assurance and governance frameworks rather than treating it as a standalone function. By linking digital risk management tools with performance indicators, staff appraisals, and regulatory reporting requirements, organisations create integrated systems that reinforce accountability and learning. This systemic approach reduces fragmentation and elevates risk assessment from a bureaucratic task to a core element of care excellence.

Furthermore, promoting a positive risk culture within organisations amplifies the benefits of technology. When staff feel supported to report risks without fear of blame and perceive risk assessment as a collaborative, value-driven activity, engagement with digital tools improves. Transparent communication about the purposes and outcomes of technology use builds trust and motivation. Recognising and celebrating examples where technology-assisted risk management has prevented harm encourages further adoption and innovation.

Looking ahead, advancements in virtual and augmented reality may provide immersive training environments for risk assessment, enabling practitioners to simulate complex scenarios safely and refine their decision-making skills. Similarly, enhanced interoperability standards may allow diverse digital systems to communicate seamlessly, creating comprehensive ecosystems that support holistic risk management across health and social care networks.

In conclusion, the challenges of risk assessment in health and social care, from accurate hazard identification to timely, consistent documentation, are significant but increasingly surmountable through thoughtful application of technology. Software, apps, and digital tracking methods, when strategically implemented and supported by robust training and cultural change, can transform risk assessment from a cumbersome obligation into a dynamic, integrated, and user-friendly process. This transformation not only improves safety and compliance but also empowers professionals and service users alike, fostering environments where risks are managed intelligently and dignity and independence are preserved. As technology continues to evolve, it will be essential for care organisations to remain adaptive, reflective, and collaborative, ensuring that digital tools serve as enablers of safer, higher-quality care, rather than barriers.

Training and Professional Development

Training Programmes

In the dynamic and multifaceted environments of health and social care, continuous professional development through comprehensive training programmes is an indispensable cornerstone for cultivating competence and confidence in risk assessment and management. The landscape of risk is ever-changing, influenced by emerging health threats, evolving legislative frameworks, technological advancements, and the diverse needs of service users. Consequently, training programmes are designed not merely as one-off instructional events but as ongoing, layered processes that embed reflective practice, facilitate skill acquisition, and promote a culture of safety and empowerment within care settings.

The array of training available encompasses a broad spectrum, tailored to meet the varying demands placed upon care providers, managers, and regulatory professionals alike. At the foundational level, induction training introduces newly appointed staff to the core principles of risk assessment, familiarising them with key concepts such as the differentiation between hazard and risk, the significance of person-centred approaches, and basic legislative imperatives such as the Health and Safety at Work Act 1974 and the Care Quality Commission's regulatory standards. This initial exposure equips staff with the fundamental vocabulary and mindset essential for safe practice and sets the stage for deeper engagement.

Building upon this, intermediate training modules delve into practical methodologies and procedural competencies. These sessions typically employ case studies, role-playing, and scenario-based learning to foster critical thinking and decision-making skills necessary for real-world applications. Care providers learn to conduct detailed hazard identification, apply risk rating tools such as risk matrices, and evaluate the effectiveness of control measures across various care contexts. The participatory nature of such programmes is crucial, inviting attendees to discuss dilemmas, reflect on past incidents, and collaboratively devise tailored management strategies that honour service users' individuality while ensuring safety. This collaborative learning environment not only enhances knowledge retention but also promotes a culture of shared responsibility.

Advanced training offerings further expand upon specialised areas such as dynamic risk assessments, safeguarding vulnerable individuals, managing complex medication regimes, and navigating mental health risks. These programmes often incorporate the latest research findings, technological tools, and legislative updates to maintain currency. For instance, workshops may explore the use of digital risk assessment platforms that streamline documentation and reporting or introduce innovative person-centred frameworks that balance autonomy with protection. Managers and team leaders frequently benefit from leadership-focused training that emphasises risk governance, legal accountability, and strategic oversight, thereby enhancing their capacity to foster compliance and cultivate environments in which staff feel supported in raising concerns and engaging in positive risk-taking. Such courses often integrate elements of coaching and mentorship, reinforcing the link between knowledge dissemination and practical support.

Moreover, the development of specialist qualifications, such as Diplomas or Certificates in Risk Management within Health and Social Care, provides structured pathways for ambitious practitioners seeking to deepen their expertise and influence organisational practices. These formal qualifications, accredited by professional bodies, offer comprehensive curricula that cover risk theory, ethical considerations, multidisciplinary collaboration, and quality assurance processes. By achieving such credentials, individuals not only elevate their own professional standing but also enhance the reputation and safety culture of their employing organisations.

Integral to all these training programmes is the emphasis on reflective practice, a vital mechanism through which practitioners continuously examine their own experiences, challenges, and outcomes in managing risk. Reflective sessions often accompany training workshops, encouraging participants to critically appraise their assumptions, consider alternative perspectives, and identify areas for improvement. This reflective component is essential in fostering adaptive learning, ensuring that risk assessment does not remain a static checklist but evolves through ongoing insight and responsiveness to changing contexts.

Accessibility and inclusivity within training programmes are also pivotal. Recognising the diverse backgrounds, roles, and learning preferences of health and social care staff, training is increasingly offered through blended learning formats that combine face-to-face instruction, e-learning modules, webinars, and interactive digital resources. This flexibility accommodates shift patterns, geographical dispersal, and varying levels of technological proficiency, making learning opportunities more equitable. Additionally, bespoke sessions tailored to specific service user groups, such as older adults, individuals with learning disabilities, or mental health service users, enhance relevance and applicability, ensuring that risk management strategies are appropriately sensitive and effective.

Beyond formal training events, the concept of a learning organisation underpins an effective risk assessment culture. Organisations are encouraged to embed continuous professional development as a strategic priority, facilitating regular refresher courses, reflective supervision, and peer learning forums. Such environments encourage the sharing of 'lessons learned' from incident reports and near-misses, promoting transparency and a proactive stance toward risk mitigation. The role of trainers and facilitators is therefore not confined to knowledge transmission but also extends to mentorship and culture-building, nurturing an ethos in which staff feel valued, informed, and empowered to act confidently.

Frequent updates to legislation, policies, and best practice guidance necessitate ongoing training refreshers to maintain compliance and align with evolving standards. For example, changes in safeguarding laws or infection control protocols require tailored briefing sessions that ensure all staff are conversant with their responsibilities and procedural adjustments. These updates may be delivered via succinct briefings, interactive online courses, or integrated into team meetings, fostering timely and practical dissemination. This dynamic approach reduces complacency and supports care providers in adapting swiftly to emerging challenges.

Another crucial dimension of training programmes involves equipping staff to utilise documentation and reporting systems effectively. Given that accurate record-keeping is essential for legal compliance, incident analysis, and multi-agency communication, training often incorporates workshops on maintaining comprehensive risk logs, completing reporting forms, and understanding whistleblowing mechanisms. Mastery of these administrative aspects enhances accountability and ensures that vital information informs service planning and safeguarding measures.

Notably, training must also address the emotional and psychological toll of risk management in care settings. Caring for vulnerable individuals and managing situations fraught with uncertainty and potential harm can provoke stress, anxiety, or moral distress among staff. Consequently, many training programmes incorporate components on self-care strategies, resilience building, and recognising signs of burnout. These elements acknowledge that a healthy, supported workforce is better positioned to make sound risk judgments and sustain compassionate practice. Peer support networks, facilitated by trained supervisors or counsellors, complement formal training in fostering wellbeing.

In addition, involvement of service users and carers in training design and delivery is an increasingly embraced practice that enriches learning experiences. By hearing firsthand accounts and perspectives, care providers gain a deeper appreciation of how risk is experienced and negotiated in daily life. This participatory approach reinforces the imperative of person-centred risk management, grounding theoretical learning in real human context and promoting empathetic, respectful care approaches.

In recent years, technological innovations have expanded the scope and accessibility of risk assessment training. Virtual reality simulations offer immersive environments where practitioners can safely rehearse responses to challenging situations, such as managing aggressive behaviour or responding to emergency evacuations. These advanced tools enhance experiential learning, enabling repeated practice and immediate feedback. Similarly, mobile applications deliver on-demand resources, reminders, and prompts to support in-situ decision-making, bridging the gap between training sessions and practical application.

Ensuring quality and effectiveness within training programmes involves rigorous evaluation mechanisms. Feedback from participants, competency assessments, and outcome monitoring help identify strengths and areas for enhancement. This evidence-informed approach supports continuous curriculum refinement, ensuring content remains relevant, engaging, and aligned with contemporary risks and care standards. Moreover, successful completion of training is often linked to appraisal processes and career progression, reinforcing its value and incentivising participation.

Ultimately, the investment in diverse and ongoing training opportunities reflects an organisation's commitment to safeguarding not only service users but also its workforce. By fostering a culture where learning is continuous, reflective, and embedded within everyday practice, health and social care providers can navigate the complexities of risk with assurance and ethical clarity. This holistic approach equips professionals at all levels to balance safety with dignity, statutory compliance with empowerment, and vigilance with innovation, ensuring that risk management truly makes a difference in the quality of care delivered.

Reflective Practice

In the ever-evolving landscape of health and social care, where risks are dynamic and the stakes incredibly high, the ability to engage in reflective practice emerges as a cornerstone of professional excellence and safety. Reflective practice, in its essence, is not merely a bureaucratic tick-box or a momentary pause in the busy routine of caregiving it embodies a deep, continuous process of self-examination and critical thinking that fuels meaningful improvements in risk management skills. As professionals in this field, our journey does not end with mastering formal training modules or complying with regulatory frameworks; rather, it is an ongoing voyage in which reflection transforms experiences, mistakes, and successes alike into enduring lessons that elevate the quality and safety of care provision.

At the heart of reflective practice lies an intrinsic commitment to continuous professional development (CPD), an indispensable ingredient for maintaining competence amid the complexity and unpredictability typical of health and social environments. As care landscapes shift with new challenges, including emerging health threats, technological advancements, and evolving legislation, stagnation in knowledge and skills inevitably translates into increased vulnerability to risks. Reflective practice serves as a dynamic bridge connecting theoretical knowledge and real-world application, enabling professionals to evaluate the outcomes of their decisions, actions, and interactions in context. By systematically considering what went well, what could have been done differently, and critical insights into the underlying assumptions or biases that influence risk perception, practitioners unlock a nuanced understanding of their practice's impact on both service users and themselves.

Within risk management specifically, reflective practice offers profound benefits beyond the confines of risk assessment checklists or policy documents. It invites health and social care workers to critically analyse how risks are identified, assessed, and mitigated in diverse scenarios, whether routine or extraordinary, and to explore the interplay between organisational procedures, personal judgment, and collaborative dynamics. For example, a moving and handling risk assessment may initially appear straightforward, but reflection may reveal subtle contextual factors such as environmental nuances, communication gaps among staff, or the unique preferences and capacities of the service user that influence risk outcomes. This reflective scrutiny leads to more tailored, encompassing risk management strategies rather than relying exclusively on generic protocols. It encourages a mindset that embraces uncertainty cautiously yet positively, fostering adaptive risk-taking that supports empowerment and dignity without compromising safety.

Importantly, reflective practice nourishes an ethical dimension in risk management by magnifying awareness of professional responsibilities, moral dilemmas, and safeguarding imperatives. When professionals pause to contemplate ethically fraught situations such as balancing autonomy against protection, they cultivate a sharper sensitivity to the complexities inherent in care decisions. This heightened ethical consciousness, reinforced through guided reflection sessions or peer discussions, enhances judgment and confidence, ultimately contributing to more compassionate and just care environments. Moreover, reflection promotes humility and openness to learning, vital antidotes to complacency or defensive attitudes that can hinder safety culture.

Embedding reflective practice into the daily routine involves deliberate strategies and support systems within organisations. Formal avenues such as structured debriefings following incidents or near misses, mentorship programs, and reflective supervision create safe spaces for candid dialogue and shared learning. These forums not only bolster individual growth but also stimulate collective awareness and improvement, reinforcing a culture that values transparent communication and accountability. Informal reflection, equally important, may transpire in moments of quiet contemplation after a challenging shift or through journaling, enabling practitioners to articulate feelings, capture insights, and process complex emotions that influence decision-making under pressure.

Training programs further enable reflective practice by equipping professionals with conceptual frameworks and tools to analyse their experiences critically and constructively. Models such as Gibbs' Reflective Cycle or the Schön reflective practitioner paradigm offer structured pathways for systematically dissecting events, fostering deeper comprehension over superficial recall. Through exercises that encourage the identification of emotional responses, the exploration of alternative actions, and the development of future action plans, these programs build both reflective capacity and risk-assessment acumen, essential for proficient care delivery. Coupled with ongoing education on evolving legal requirements, best-practice guidelines, and emerging risk factors, such integration of reflective methods ensures that care providers remain agile and informed in their risk-management approaches.

Reflection also plays a pivotal role in enhancing collaboration among multi-disciplinary teams and external agencies involved in health and social care. By openly sharing reflections on risk incidents, professionals contribute to a richer collective knowledge base, aiding the identification of systemic issues or recurring hazards that may elude solitary scrutiny. This openness fosters trust and cohesiveness, qualities indispensable when coordinating complex care plans or responding to safeguarding concerns. Moreover, reflective dialogues across disciplines facilitate appreciation of differing perspectives and expertise, enriching risk assessments with holistic insights that might otherwise remain siloed within individual roles.

The benefits of reflective practice extend beyond the immediate professional domain, impacting broader organisational safety culture and ultimately the experiences and outcomes for service users. When reflection is genuinely valued and integrated, it signals a commitment to learning and improvement that transcends compliance and touches on the core of care quality. It empowers practitioners to recognise and navigate the tension between managing harm and promoting independence, creatively and sensitively, in line with the ethos of person-centred care. As a result, risk assessments become living documents, responsive to changing needs and informed by ongoing experiential learning rather than static protocols.

Nevertheless, embedding reflective practice into risk management requires deliberate effort to overcome potential barriers. Time constraints, workload pressures, and a lack of reflective skills or confidence can impede practitioners from engaging meaningfully with reflection. Additionally, organisational cultures that prioritise fault-finding over learning may discourage openness or foster fear of blame, stifling reflective honesty. To counter these obstacles, leadership must champion reflective practice explicitly as a valued element of professional development and risk governance, allocating resources, training, and protected time accordingly. Emphasising the formative nature of reflection as a tool for growth rather than judgment helps build psychological safety, encouraging staff at all levels to share insights and learn without fear.

Furthermore, technology increasingly supports the integration of reflective practice and risk management. Digital platforms for recording risk assessments, incident reports, and reflective notes enable streamlined access and pattern recognition that might be imperceptible through paper-based methods. These tools can prompt reflective prompts, facilitate peer feedback, and document learning trajectories, fostering an evidence-informed culture of continuous improvement. Still, technology complements, not replaces, the human factors of empathy, critical thinking, and dialogue essential for authentic reflective practice.

In summary, reflective practice is a vital mechanism for health and social care professionals to enhance their risk management skills, integrating knowledge, experience, ethics, and collaboration into a cohesive approach to safer, person-centred care. By embracing reflection as a continuous and deliberate process, practitioners deepen their understanding of complex risks, refine their judgments, and adapt innovatively to ever-changing care environments. Organisations that embed a reflective culture signal a genuine commitment to professional growth, transparency, and the safeguarding of excellence. Through formal training, supportive supervision, peer collaboration, and mindful individual practice, reflection becomes an empowering journey transforming challenges into opportunities, mistakes into lessons, and risk management from a procedural exercise into a dynamic, thoughtful practice that truly makes a difference for everyone involved.

Evaluating Training Effectiveness

Evaluating training effectiveness within health and social care settings represents a pivotal component of ensuring continuous professional development and maintaining high standards of care delivery. The dynamic nature of health and social care environments, coupled with evolving legislation and practice standards, necessitates that training programs are not only delivered but also rigorously assessed for their actual impact on knowledge, skills, attitudes, and ultimately, patient and service user outcomes. Without such evaluation, training risks becoming a perfunctory exercise, an obligatory tick-box activity devoid of meaningful improvement or tangible benefit. Thus, the methodology of evaluating training effectiveness must be approached with as much seriousness and intentionality as the design and implementation of the training itself, anchoring it firmly in both theoretical underpinnings and practical realities.

One foundational approach to assessing training effectiveness is Kirkpatrick's Four-Level Training Evaluation Model, which provides a systematic framework for evaluating multiple dimensions of learning interventions. The first level, reaction, measures how participants respond to the training: their engagement, satisfaction, and perceived relevance. This often involves immediate feedback collected through questionnaires or informal discussions, providing valuable, albeit subjective, insight into learners' experiences. While understanding participants' reactions is important for ensuring training enjoyment and motivation, it only scratches the surface when evaluating true effectiveness. A training session that is enjoyable but devoid of substantive content or practical application fails to achieve its intended outcomes.

Progressing beyond reaction, the second level, learning, examines the extent to which trainees acquire the intended knowledge, skills, and attitudes. This level transfers evaluative efforts from feelings to measurable cognitive and behavioural changes. Pre- and post-training assessments, quizzes, practical demonstrations, and reflective exercises are common tools for assessing learning. In health and social care, this might include testing knowledge of risk assessment principles, demonstrating competency in hazard identification, or applying new protocols through simulated case studies. It is crucial that these assessments are designed thoughtfully to mirror real-world scenarios and challenge learners in authentic ways. Nonetheless, learning validation at this level still does not guarantee that new knowledge is enacted in the work environment or transferred to daily practice, hence the necessity of further levels of evaluation.

The third level, behaviour, scrutinises whether the learning has been translated into changes in practice. It involves observing, measuring, and confirming that trainees are effectively applying their newly acquired competencies when performing their roles. This level is notoriously challenging to assess due to the complexities of care environments, varying workplace cultures, and external factors such as staffing levels and resource availability. Methods for evaluating behaviour change include direct observation during work, peer assessments, supervisor feedback, and performance appraisals. Additionally, reflective practice is particularly significant here, as continual self-assessment encourages care providers to critically examine their behaviours, embrace accountability, and identify areas for improvement. Establishing mechanisms that support reflection, such as journals, mentorship conversations, or structured supervision sessions, is intrinsic to embedding behaviour change and sustaining professional growth.

Finally, the fourth and most impactful level in Kirkpatrick's model involves results, the ultimate evaluation of whether training positively influences organisational goals, enhances service user safety, and contributes to improved care quality. This may encompass metrics such as reduced incidence of accidents or errors, higher compliance with health and safety regulations, improved safeguarding outcomes, or elevated patient satisfaction scores. These outcome indicators provide strong evidence of training success but are difficult to attribute exclusively to individual training due to numerous intervening variables. Consequently, organisations must adopt a holistic approach, integrating training evaluation with broader quality and safety monitoring systems to capture nuanced impacts.

While Kirkpatrick's model remains a cornerstone, contemporary frameworks emphasise more nuanced, iterative approaches to evaluation, especially in health and social care, where complexity and ethical considerations abound. Constructivist theories propose that adult learning is experiential, social, and context-dependent; thus, evaluation processes must capture the richness of learners' application in real-world contexts rather than mere rote acquisition. Appreciative inquiry, for instance, invites stakeholders to collaboratively identify strengths, envision ideal practices, and design improvements, fostering a positive, forward-looking culture around training efficacy.

Crucially, evaluating training effectiveness aligns closely with the principle of continuous professional development (CPD) that is foundational in health and social care. CPD encourages practitioners to view learning as an ongoing journey rather than a one-off event. Effective evaluation feeds this process by identifying gaps in knowledge or application, illuminating areas for further learning, and acknowledging achievement, thereby reinforcing motivation and professional identity. Integrating evaluation results into CPD planning creates a feedback loop in which each training iteration is refined, and practitioners remain aligned with best practice and legislative changes.

In practice, a multi-method approach yields richer, more reliable data on training effectiveness. Combining quantitative techniques such as tests and surveys with qualitative methods such as interviews, focus groups, and reflective narratives provides a multidimensional understanding. For example, quantitative data may reveal statistically significant improvements in knowledge scores, while qualitative feedback captures contextual factors influencing application, such as team dynamics or organisational culture. Organisational leaders and managers play a vital role in facilitating these evaluations by encouraging open dialogue, allocating time and resources for reflective practice, and genuinely valuing employee input rather than treating it superficially.

An essential aspect often overlooked in training evaluation is the role of service users and carers in providing feedback on the impacts of staff training. Engaging those directly affected by health and social care services enriches the evaluation by introducing perspectives grounded in lived experience. Their observations on staff competence, empathy, and responsiveness can signal whether training has effectively translated into better care relationships and outcomes. This participatory approach reinforces person-centred values and strengthens trust between service users and providers.

Moreover, in the evolving landscape of health and social care, technological advancements have introduced new modalities for evaluating training effectiveness. Digital platforms permit the collection of real-time data through e-learning assessments, virtual simulations, and adaptive learning systems that tailor content to individual needs. The use of mobile applications enables immediate feedback and reflection prompts during or after training events. Additionally, data analytics facilitate tracking of longitudinal performance trends, identifying patterns that may not be apparent from isolated evaluations. However, technology complements but does not replace the critical human elements of evaluation, especially in interpreting complex behaviours, attitudes, and ethical decision-making processes inherent in care provision.

Sustaining improvements from training evaluation requires a culture that embraces learning and safety. It necessitates leadership commitment to acting on evaluation findings, whether that involves revising training curricula, enhancing support mechanisms such as supervision and coaching, or addressing systemic barriers that impede application. For instance, if evaluation reveals that staff struggle to conduct effective risk assessments due to time constraints or inadequate equipment, meaningful organisational changes must follow. Otherwise, evaluation risks becoming a performative act without real impact. This underscores the interconnectedness of training effectiveness with organisational climate, resource allocation, and policy priorities.

Equally important is fostering an environment that encourages open reporting of challenges encountered during training uptake without fear of blame or reprisal. Psychological safety enables practitioners to share difficulties, ask questions, and propose innovations that improve care standards. Evaluating and responding to training effectiveness within such a supportive context accelerates learning and motivates continuous improvement. It reflects an understanding that human error and uncertainty are part of care processes and that learning from these is more constructive than punitive approaches.

Reflective practice also acts as a critical internal thermometer for evaluating training outcomes at the individual level. By engaging in structured reflection before, during, and after training activities, practitioners can articulate learning objectives, monitor progress, and critically assess the transfer of knowledge into practice. Models such as Gibbs' Reflective Cycle or Schön's Reflection-in-Action encourage thoughtful analysis of experiences, emotions, and outcomes, leading to deeper insights and enhanced competence. Embedding reflective practice into the workplace culture supports not only personal development but collective learning when facilitated through team discussions and peer support.

In evaluating training effectiveness, attention must also be given to the differential impacts across workforce diversity. Health and social care settings employ individuals with varied backgrounds, education levels, experiences, and learning styles. A one-size-fits-all evaluation approach risks marginalising some voices and masking inequities in learning outcomes. Tailoring evaluation tools to be culturally sensitive, accessible, and inclusive fosters fairness and a richer understanding. Furthermore, recognising that staff at different career stages have distinct developmental needs and responses to training informs differentiated evaluation strategies, ensuring relevance and engagement.

Finally, the iterative cycle of planning, delivering, evaluating, and refining training encapsulates a philosophy of lifelong learning essential to health and social care professionalism. Effective evaluation is not a singular endpoint but an ongoing dialogue between learners, educators, managers, and stakeholders, continuously adapting to changing needs, evidence, and contexts. This iterative process positions training not merely as a compliance activity but as a dynamic lever for excellence in care quality, safeguarding, and service user empowerment. By rigorously evaluating and improving training programs, health and social care providers demonstrate their unwavering commitment to competence, safety, and dignity, ultimately making a positive difference in the lives they touch every day.

Future Trends in Health and Social Care Risk Management

Emerging Risks

In the rapidly evolving landscape of health and social care, the concept of risk is far from static; it continually shifts in response to societal changes, technological advances, regulatory updates, and the dynamic nature of service users' needs. Emerging risks pose a unique challenge to care providers, who must remain vigilant and adaptable to protect the well-being of those in their charge. The very fabric of health and social care delivery is being reshaped by factors that once seemed distant or non-existent. These novel challenges range from the advent of complex technologies and digital systems to the changing demographics and health profiles of populations served, all converging to create a multidimensional risk environment that demands fresh approaches to assessment and management.

One of the foremost sources of emerging risk is the proliferation of technology in care settings. The adoption of digital health records, telecare, wearable monitoring devices, and even artificial intelligence-driven decision-support tools has created unprecedented opportunities to enhance service delivery. However, alongside these innovations come vulnerabilities related to data security, privacy breaches, and system failures. Care providers must now navigate the intersection of clinical best practice and cyber safety, ensuring that sensitive personal information remains confidential against threats of hacking or accidental disclosure. The complexity of safeguarding digital assets creates a parallel risk landscape that is not purely clinical or physical but equally critical. When electronic systems fail, whether through technical glitches or cyberattacks, the consequences can ripple through care provision, disrupting medication administration, delaying emergency responses, or compromising essential communication pathways among multidisciplinary teams.

Alongside technological risks, the demographic and epidemiological shifts influencing health and social care present novel challenges. The ageing population, coupled with the increasing prevalence of multi-morbidity, where individuals live with multiple chronic conditions, complicates traditional risk assessment frameworks. Conditions such as dementia, frailty, and mental health disorders require more nuanced evaluations that balance physical safety with psychological well-being and autonomy. This complexity is heightened by the diversity of service users, whose cultural backgrounds, communication needs, and personal preferences must be factored into meaningful risk assessments. The need to deliver personalised care that respects individual values while managing safety often leads to tensions that care providers must carefully navigate. For example, encouraging independence for a person with mild cognitive impairment may introduce fall risks, yet overly restrictive practices erode quality of life. Such dilemmas reflect a shifting paradigm where risk is not solely about prevention but also about understanding and managing acceptable levels of uncertainty in pursuit of dignity and choice.

Regulatory frameworks themselves are evolving in response to societal demands for enhanced transparency, accountability, and safety in care settings. Recent policy changes emphasise not only risk prevention but also the active promotion of positive risk-taking, recognising that some degree of risk is inherent and even beneficial for personal growth and independence. This necessitates a cultural shift within organisations that have traditionally leaned toward risk aversion. Embedding this ethos requires care providers to develop skills in dynamic risk assessment and collaborative decision-making, involving service users and families as active partners. However, aligning practice with new standards often presents logistical and educational challenges, particularly in under-resourced settings or among staff unfamiliar with the philosophical underpinnings of positive risk-taking. The constant evolution of statutory guidance demands continual professional development and organisational agility to ensure compliance and uphold safety without stifling empowerment.

Innovation in safety practices is another frontier shaping emerging risks. Advances such as simulation training, virtual reality environments for skill-building, and sophisticated incident reporting systems contribute significantly to proactive risk management. These tools can uncover latent hazards and facilitate experiential learning, allowing care workers to rehearse responses to uncommon or complex situations in controlled settings. The integration of human factors science further enriches understanding by examining how cognitive, social, and environmental elements interact to influence errors and near misses. Despite their promise, such innovations require careful implementation and evaluation to avoid unintended consequences, such as increased workload or technological dependence that may overshadow essential human judgment. Balancing cutting-edge safety methodologies with practical realities remains an ongoing balancing act, demanding leadership commitment and adaptive strategies.

Perhaps one of the most transformative developments in risk assessment is the expanding role of data analytics and predictive modelling. The abundance of data generated within health and social care, from electronic health records to sensor data in smart homes, offers unprecedented potential to identify patterns and forecast risks before adverse events occur. Sophisticated algorithms can analyse complex variables, revealing correlations that might elude traditional clinical intuition. For instance, predictive tools might highlight early warning signs for falls or medication errors, allowing timely intervention. This data-driven approach shifts the paradigm toward preventative care and individualised risk profiles, fostering more precise, evidence-based decision-making. However, reliance on analytics also raises questions about data quality, algorithmic bias, and ethical considerations around consent and transparency. Care providers must develop competencies not only in interpreting data outputs but also in understanding the limitations and ensuring that technology complements rather than replaces frontline clinical judgment.

Social determinants of health are increasingly recognised as key contributors to emerging risks within care contexts. Factors such as housing instability, social isolation, poverty, and systemic inequalities profoundly influence individuals' vulnerability and access to services. Addressing risks associated with these determinants requires holistic approaches that extend beyond immediate clinical concerns. Collaboration with community services, advocacy for policy interventions, and culturally competent care become essential components of risk management. Care providers must expand their scope to include social risk factors, integrating them into assessments to develop comprehensive care plans. This broader perspective aligns with the move towards person-centred and integrated care models but introduces complexities in information sharing, resource allocation, and interagency coordination. Emerging risks, therefore, are not merely clinical or operational but embedded within wider societal structures that require multifaceted strategies.

Environmental and public health threats represent another evolving sphere of risk that affects health and social care delivery. Climate change, pandemics, and antibiotic resistance exemplify challenges with far-reaching consequences. Extreme weather events threaten the stability of infrastructure and disrupt care pathways, while infectious disease outbreaks demand rapid adaptation of protocols and heightened infection control measures. The Covid-19 pandemic is a poignant example of how a global health crisis can redefine risk priorities overnight, necessitating unprecedented collaboration, reassessment of protocols, and deployment of new technologies such as remote consultations. The pandemic also highlighted vulnerabilities in staffing, supply chains, and mental health support, underscoring the interconnectedness of risk factors. Care providers must build resilience and contingency planning into their risk management frameworks to navigate these unpredictable yet impactful threats.

It is also crucial to acknowledge the human element as a source and mitigator of emerging risks. Workforce challenges such as recruitment shortages, burnout, and varied skill levels affect the consistency and quality of risk assessment and management. Staff under pressure may miss critical cues or avoid comprehensive documentation, inadvertently increasing risk exposure. At the same time, fostering a workplace culture that encourages open communication, shared learning from incidents, and psychological safety can significantly reduce errors and enhance risk awareness. Leadership plays a pivotal role in shaping such environments, promoting continuous professional development, and valuing frontline insights. Additionally, embracing diversity and inclusion within teams can enhance problem-solving and sensitivity toward varied risk factors encountered by diverse populations. Emerging risks thus intersect with organisational culture and human factors in ways that must be deliberately addressed.

Furthermore, ethical considerations are gaining prominence as digital and clinical innovations reshape care pathways. Issues surrounding consent, autonomy, confidentiality, and the equitable distribution of resources require constant vigilance. As care providers harness technologies and complex data tools, they must balance innovation with respect for human rights and ethical standards. This is especially pertinent when considering predictive analytics that might label individuals as 'high-risk' and potentially affect access to services or stigma. Transparency, participatory decision-making, and clear governance structures are essential to navigating these tensions. Similarly, ethical implications of positive risk-taking must be continually examined to avoid compromising safety while supporting independence. Emerging risks, therefore, invite ongoing reflection not only on procedural adaptations but also on the underlying moral frameworks that guide care.

In responding to these multifaceted emerging risks, health and social care providers must adopt a forward-looking, adaptive posture. This calls for investments in training that enhance digital literacy, ethical reasoning, and collaborative problem-solving. Encouraging a learning organisation culture where innovation is embraced yet critically appraised will help integrate new tools and methodologies effectively. Interprofessional collaboration, both within care teams and across agencies, must be strengthened to share knowledge, resources, and best practices in the face of evolving challenges. The integration of service user voices is also paramount, ensuring that risk management strategies reflect lived experience and preferences. Policymakers and regulators, in turn, should support flexible frameworks that accommodate innovation while safeguarding core principles of care quality and safety.

Ultimately, confronting emerging risks in health and social care requires embracing complexity and uncertainty with informed confidence. The landscape will continue to shift as technology advances, populations change, and societal expectations evolve. Providers who cultivate agility, critical thinking, and ethical sensitivity can transform these challenges into opportunities for improving care outcomes, enhancing safety, and promoting dignity. By proactively engaging with emerging risks, anticipating them, learning from them, and innovating, health and social care practitioners thoughtfully will not only protect those they serve but also contribute to shaping resilient and responsive care systems fit for the future.

Innovations in Practice

In the ever-evolving landscape of health and social care, innovations in risk assessment and management have become not only desirable but indispensable for delivering safe and effective care in a complex world. The traditional paradigms of risk assessment, while foundational, must continuously adapt to the evolving nature of risks that emerge from rapid technological advances, shifting policy environments, and an increasingly interconnected, data-rich ecosystem. Today's health and social care arenas face an expanding array of challenges that require fresh thinking, new tools, and innovative procedural approaches to not only identify and control hazards but to anticipate and prevent them. This subchapter delves into the dynamic interplay of technological and procedural innovations that are reshaping how risk is managed, spotlighting the transformative impact of data analytics, digital tools, adaptive policies, and multidisciplinary collaboration on improving the quality and safety of care.

Health and social care settings have traditionally relied on manual, paper-based, and linear methodologies to identify risks, record findings, and monitor mitigations. While these have served their purpose, the complexity and pace of service delivery today demand more agile, responsive, and integrated approaches. Innovations driven by technology have introduced smarter ways to capture and analyse risk-related data in real time, enabling practitioners and managers to make proactive decisions. For instance, electronic risk management systems have replaced cumbersome paper documentation, providing digital dashboards where care providers can input hazard observations, receive automated alerts, and track the effectiveness of control measures. This shift alone represents a monumental improvement in efficiency and accuracy, allowing for the aggregation of data across teams and departments, revealing patterns and potential systemic issues that would otherwise remain hidden.

One prominent innovation that has revolutionised risk management in recent years is the application of advanced data analytics and artificial intelligence (AI). In many ways, these tools transcend traditional risk assessment by enabling predictive analytics to forecast risks before they manifest, using historical and real-time data trends. Data from electronic health records, incident reports, sensor devices, and even social determinants of health can be integrated and analysed using sophisticated algorithms to detect subtle signals of emerging risks. For example, predictive models can identify individuals at higher risk of falls or medication errors by analysing multiple interacting variables simultaneously, thereby empowering care providers to intervene with tailored prevention strategies. This shift from reactive to proactive risk management exemplifies innovation not just as a matter of technology but as a fundamental reshaping of the philosophy of care.

Technology's role is equally critical in managing evolving risks arising from increasingly complex care environments and diverse service users. The rise of home and community-based care introduces new layers of unpredictability compared to controlled institutional settings, necessitating portable, user-friendly tools for dynamic risk assessments. Mobile applications now allow practitioners to conduct and update assessments on the go, incorporating multimedia inputs such as photos, voice notes, and geolocation data to enrich the contextual understanding of risks. Such tools enhance communication among multidisciplinary teams by providing shared, up-to-date risk profiles, ensuring everyone remains informed and aligned in their interventions. These innovations reflect an important trend towards person-centred risk management where real-time data and technology converge to support individuals' safety without compromising their autonomy.

Beyond data and digital tools, procedural innovations continue to define best practices in risk management. The concept of dynamic risk assessment, which recognises that risk levels fluctuate in response to changing circumstances, has become a core principle, especially in emergency care, mental health, and community care settings. Instead of fixed, static assessments completed at regular intervals, dynamic assessments employ flexible, ongoing evaluation that encourages practitioners to remain vigilant and responsive throughout their interactions. Innovations in training and clinical supervision incorporate simulated scenarios, decision-support algorithms, and team-based reflective practices to better equip frontline staff with the skills and judgment required for such fluid risk management. The integration of simulation-based learning has allowed care providers to experience a wide range of risk scenarios in controlled environments, enhancing their ability to make rapid, informed decisions under pressure while ensuring safety.

Complementing these technological and procedural advances are notable shifts in policy frameworks and regulatory guidelines that reflect contemporary understandings of risk and safety. Over the past decade, there has been a growing emphasis on positive risk-taking, a paradigm that balances the imperative to protect service users with the imperative to respect their rights and promote autonomy. This has prompted re-examination of existing policies that were traditionally risk-averse, encouraging more nuanced approaches that foster empowerment while maintaining vigilance. Innovations in policy now integrate person-centred risk assessments as standard practice, recognising that safeguarding is not solely about restriction but about enabling meaningful participation. This recalibration of risk culture within organisations requires not only new frameworks but also leadership that models openness to innovation and continuous learning. Regulatory agencies have similarly adapted their standards to expect evidence of dynamic, collaborative, and data-informed risk management processes, placing innovation at the heart of compliance.

The integration of technology and policy-driven innovation naturally leads to enhanced collaboration and communication among care stakeholders. In complex care scenarios, risk management benefits immensely from transparent data-sharing platforms and multi-agency networks that break down silos between health, social care, mental health, and community services. Innovations such as secure cloud-based systems, interoperable electronic records, and mobile communication apps have made it feasible for teams separated by geography and disciplines to work synchronously. This collaborative environment fosters collective risk intelligence, where shared insights help anticipate and mitigate risks more comprehensively. Case conferences, virtual multi-disciplinary team meetings, and joint risk registers are examples of processes enhanced by technology and procedural reform. Such innovations not only improve risk management outcomes but also build resilience within care systems, enabling faster adaptation to emerging threats such as pandemics or demographic shifts.

A compelling example of innovation in practice is seen in the use of wearable technologies and the Internet of Things (IoT) to enhance safety monitoring for vulnerable populations. Devices that continuously monitor vital signs, movement patterns, and environmental conditions can detect deviations that indicate risk events such as falls, dehydration, or agitation. By transmitting alerts to care staff or family members, these technological innovations provide an extra layer of protection while supporting individuals' independence. Moreover, the data collected over time can feed into risk models, further refining personalised care planning. Although these advances raise ethical and privacy considerations that require careful governance, their potential to transform risk assessment practice is profound.

Furthermore, the emergence of telehealth and remote monitoring technologies has reshaped how many services manage risk, particularly in rural or underserved areas. Teleconsultations reduce risks associated with travel and exposure to infectious diseases, while remote monitoring enables continuous oversight of chronic conditions. This layered innovation model combines technological advances and process redesign, allowing practitioners to remain vigilant about patients' well-being without requiring constant physical presence. These developments raise further questions and opportunities related to digital literacy among service users and staff, access equity, and the evolving roles of care providers. Nonetheless, the confluence of technology and reimagined care pathways exemplifies how risk management can expand beyond narrowly defined settings to adapt to modern realities.

In addition to technology-driven tools and procedural shifts, innovation in risk management also embraces evolving methodologies such as human factors engineering and systems thinking. Recognising that most errors and hazards do not result from individual failings but from systemic issues, health and social care organisations now incorporate these interdisciplinary approaches to analyse risk comprehensively. Human factors focus on designing environments, workflows, and technologies that accommodate human limitations and leverage strengths, thereby reducing the likelihood of errors. Systems thinking encourages understanding risk within the broader organisational and social context, prompting interventions that address root causes rather than symptoms. Innovations in training and leadership development integrate these perspectives, cultivating a workforce equipped to navigate complexity and design safer care systems.

Data privacy, security, and ethical considerations simultaneously emerge as critical themes amid this wave of innovation. The vast amounts of personal and sensitive data collected for risk analysis must be safeguarded through robust cybersecurity practices and transparent governance. Innovations in data anonymisation, consent management, and user control over personal information reflect ongoing efforts to balance the benefits of data-driven risk management with individual rights. Ethical frameworks guiding innovation emphasise the importance of equity, the avoidance of bias in algorithmic decision-making, and the assurance that new technologies serve to enhance rather than diminish the dignity and autonomy of service users. These dimensions highlight that true innovation is multi-faceted, encompassing technical capability, procedural soundness, policy alignment, and ethical integrity.

Another area of growing innovation is the development of integrated training platforms that combine e-learning, virtual reality, and augmented reality to simulate complex risk scenarios and enhance practitioner preparedness. Such immersive technologies allow learners to engage in interactive risk assessments and management exercises that replicate real-world situations without endangering actual service users. This experiential learning approach accelerates skill acquisition, fosters critical thinking, and builds confidence in decision-making under uncertain conditions. Moreover, it provides opportunities for interprofessional education, reinforcing teamwork and shared accountability in risk management. These advances represent a convergence of educational theory and technological possibilities, enhancing the capacity of health and social care workers to recognise, respond to, and mitigate risks effectively.

Significantly, innovation in risk assessment is not limited to tools and technologies but extends to cultural transformation within organisations. The adoption of open reporting cultures, where staff feel safe reporting near misses and incidents without fear of blame, represents a procedural innovation that enriches risk intelligence. Digital incident reporting systems with anonymous submission options, real-time feedback, and learning loops foster transparency and continuous improvement. Leadership plays a pivotal role in nurturing such cultures by modelling openness, investing in staff development, and incentivising innovation. This cultural evolution aligns with contemporary safety science, emphasising resilience, adaptability, and learning as cornerstones of effective risk management.

In response to emerging global challenges such as the COVID-19 pandemic, innovation in risk assessment and management has accelerated dramatically. The need for rapid risk identification, communication, and control across diverse and often overloaded care settings has led to the deployment of novel technological solutions and streamlined procedures. Mobile contact tracing apps, AI-powered resource allocation tools, and robust infection control protocols exemplify how innovation can be mobilised at scale in crises. These responses have demonstrated the value of maintaining flexible, technology-enabled infrastructure and adaptive policies capable of responding swiftly and effectively to emerging threats, lessons that will continue to inform risk practice moving forward.

Importantly, the integration of service users and their families in risk management is also evolving through innovation. Digital platforms now allow service users to actively engage with their care plans, report concerns, and participate in shared decision-making about acceptable risks and safeguarding measures. This shift from passive recipients to empowered partners reflects a broader societal movement towards transparency, personalisation, and respect for individual agency. Technological tools that facilitate communication, education, and feedback enhance this involvement while procedural innovations underpin collaborative risk assessment practices. Such approaches ensure that risk management is not a top-down imposition but a compassionate dialogue that respects the voices and lived experiences of those receiving care.

In sum, the innovations transforming risk assessment and management within health and social care are multifaceted, intertwining technological advances with procedural reforms, cultural change, policy evolution, and ethical reflection. Data analytics and AI enable more precise, predictive, and proactive interventions, while mobile and wearable technologies support dynamic, person-centred approaches. Training and leadership development empower the workforce to navigate complexity with resilience, and integrated communication platforms foster collaboration across professional and organisational boundaries. At the same time, a renewed commitment to positive risk-taking, safeguarding, and service user empowerment recalibrates the very ethos of risk management. These innovations serve as a beacon of progress in a challenging, high-stakes field, enhancing safety and quality while respecting dignity and promoting continuous learning. As health and social care continue to evolve amid demographic shifts, technological revolutions, and societal expectations, innovation in risk practice will remain a critical driver of positive change and excellence.

Data Analytics and Decision-Making

In the intricate and evolving landscape of health and social care, the capacity to anticipate and mitigate risks effectively increasingly hinges on data analytics. The traditional paradigms of risk management, often grounded in manual observation and retrospective incident reviews, are rapidly being transformed by technological advances that enable proactive, data-driven decision-making. This shift is not merely a technical upgrade but signifies a fundamental change in how risks are perceived, assessed, and controlled. Data analytics offers a dynamic toolset that empowers care providers and managers to decipher complex patterns, forecast potential hazards before they materialise, and tailor interventions with precision. At its core, this approach recognises that risk is not static but fluid, moulded continually by changes in policies, innovations in care practice, and the diverse needs of service users.

The first dimension to appreciate in leveraging data analytics for risk management is the evolving nature of the risks themselves. Health and social care contexts are characterised by a broad array of hazards, ranging from physical dangers such as falls and infections to more subtle psychosocial risks, including isolation and stress-related conditions. These risks do not exist in isolation; they intersect and fluctuate with factors such as demographic shifts, emerging diseases, and technological changes within the care environment. Data drawn from electronic health records, incident reports, sensor technologies, and even social care feedback mechanisms converge to form a comprehensive tapestry of information. Through sophisticated analytics, this rich dataset can be dissected to identify not only the frequency and severity of specific risks but also the underlying trends that signal potential escalations. For example, predictive models might analyse patterns indicating which service users are more susceptible to medication errors or which environmental factors correlate with increased falls in a particular care setting. Such insights allow for pre-emptive measures, shifting the focus from reactive crisis management to anticipatory risk aversion, thereby enhancing overall safety and quality of care.

Policy changes act as another potent driver in the continuum of risk evolution, demanding that data analytics be both agile and responsive. Health and social care policies are subject to frequent amendments, often aimed at improving service standards, safeguarding, and operational efficiency. Each policy alteration can inadvertently influence risk profiles in care settings. For example, new infection-control regulations necessitate stringent data monitoring to ensure compliance and detect early signs of lapses. Additionally, funding reforms or workforce directives may change the composition and availability of care personnel, impacting the delivery and associated risks. Data analytics platforms, when designed to integrate real-time policy updates, can automatically adjust risk assessment algorithms to reflect these external pressures. This capacity to align analytic models with the current regulatory environment ensures that risk management remains relevant and legally compliant, avoiding blind spots that could lead to adverse outcomes or sanctions.

Innovation in safety practices, fuelled by data insights, represents a third avenue for better risk management. New technologies such as wearable monitoring devices, ambient sensors, and AI-driven diagnostic tools generate continuous streams of high-fidelity data that were previously unavailable. These innovations allow for a granular understanding of a service user's condition and environment, enabling nuanced risk stratification. For instance, wearable devices can alert staff to early signs of agitation in individuals with dementia, helping prevent potential injury to both the person and caregivers. Similarly, environmental sensors can detect changes in room temperature or air quality that might elevate biological hazards, allowing prompt remedial action. By harnessing these technologies within a robust data infrastructure, care providers can move towards truly personalised risk management strategies that respect the unique circumstances of each service user. Moreover, data analytics can facilitate the evaluation and continuous improvement of these innovative safety practices, identifying areas of success and opportunities for refinement.

Central to this entire ecosystem is the role of data analytics in decision-making. Unlike traditional approaches that may rely predominantly on anecdotal evidence or periodic audits, data analytics provides a continuous, objective, and evidence-based foundation for risk management decisions. By applying statistical methods, machine learning algorithms, and data visualisation techniques, complex datasets are transformed into actionable knowledge. Decision-makers, including care providers, managers, and regulatory agents, benefit from clear insights about where risks are most pronounced, which control measures are effective, and how resources can be optimally allocated. For example, a heat map generated from risk data can highlight hotspots within a facility that require immediate attention, while trend analyses can guide strategic planning on training needs or infrastructure investment. Importantly, these analytic outputs are also valuable in communicating risk status and resource priorities across multidisciplinary teams, fostering transparency and shared accountability.

However, effectively leveraging data analytics requires health and social care organisations to develop robust data governance frameworks that safeguard privacy, ensure data quality, and promote interoperability. Given the sensitive nature of health and social care data, privacy and consent are paramount. Organisations must establish secure data handling procedures alongside clear policies on data accessibility to maintain service users' trust. At the same time, data quality, encompassing accuracy, completeness, and timeliness, is critical for deriving meaningful insights. Poor data quality can lead to misguided decisions, perpetuating rather than mitigating risk. Therefore, investment in training staff on accurate data entry and verification, alongside the deployment of user-friendly data capture tools, is necessary. Moreover, interoperability among data systems, such as electronic care records and incident reporting platforms, further enhances analytical potential by creating comprehensive, linked datasets. This integrative capacity uncovers deeper risk interrelations that isolated data points might miss.

It is also essential to recognise that data analytics should not replace professional judgement but rather augment it. The human element in health and social care remains central; data-driven insights should be interpreted within the context of individual needs and professional expertise. When combined, these elements form a powerful synergy that supports balanced risk-taking, which is pivotal to promoting independence and dignity among service users. For example, analytics might identify elevated fall risk in a service user, but a care provider's understanding of that individual's preferences, routines, and environment enables crafting tailored interventions that respect their autonomy. This balanced approach aligns seamlessly with contemporary care philosophies that view risk as a dynamic element to be managed rather than eliminated, underscoring care providers' ethical responsibility to empower service users while ensuring safety.

Importantly, the evolution of data analytics in health and social care mirrors a broader culture of continuous improvement. The iterative nature of data analysis fosters ongoing learning, in which risk assessments are regularly refined, and control measures are continually evaluated against emerging evidence. This continuous feedback loop promotes adaptive risk management, making organisations more resilient to unforeseen challenges. For instance, the outbreak of an infectious disease within a care home triggers rapid data collection and analysis on transmission patterns, enabling swift modification of infection control measures. Over time, these datasets contribute to building organisational knowledge and inform policy development and staff training in a manner grounded in real-world experience. This culture of learning, supported by robust data analytics, strengthens not only operational efficiency but also moral accountability towards service users and their families.

Furthermore, collaboration and communication among multiple stakeholders are profoundly enhanced through data analytics. Health and social care rarely operate in silos; the involvement of regulatory agencies, care providers, service users, families, and third-party organisations demands seamless information sharing and joint decision-making. Data dashboards and shared analytic platforms provide transparent and accessible means for different parties to monitor risk status and coordinate responses. For regulatory agents, data analytics facilitate oversight by providing real-time compliance monitoring and flagging areas of concern. For managers and care providers, shared data ensures consistency in applying risk control measures and enables rapid mobilisation of resources when necessary. This interconnectedness cultivates a unified approach to risk management, ensuring that all voices are heard and that interventions are cohesive and comprehensive, ultimately enhancing care quality and safeguarding.

As the health and social care sector continues to embrace digital transformation, emerging trends such as artificial intelligence, big data, and predictive analytics promise to further revolutionise risk assessment and decision-making processes. These technologies offer the prospect of even more nuanced and earlier risk identification, automated alerts, and enhanced scenario modelling, supporting foresight and strategic planning at unprecedented levels. However, their implementation must be accompanied by ethical scrutiny, user-centred design, and sustained support to ensure effective integration into daily practice. Equipping the workforce with data literacy skills, fostering a culture that is open to innovation, and ensuring inclusivity are critical to unlocking the full benefits of data analytics for risk mitigation. This future-oriented vision underscores that data analytics is not simply a tool but a transformative catalyst for safer, more responsive, and person-centred health and social care environments.

In summary, data analytics has emerged as an indispensable ally in the pursuit of effective risk assessment and management within health and social care. By enabling a sophisticated understanding of dynamic risks, accommodating policy and practice changes, fostering innovation in safety measures, and underpinning informed decision-making, data analytics profoundly reshape the landscape of care provision. Its potential to enhance collaboration, promote continuous improvement, and balance safety with dignity offers a compelling pathway toward improved outcomes for service users and care providers alike. As the sector navigates this complex and data-rich future, embracing analytical insights with professional expertise will be essential to making informed, ethical, and impactful decisions that safeguard wellbeing and empower everyone involved in care.

www.ingramcontent.com/pod-product-compliance
Lightning Source LLC
LaVergne TN
LVHW062029051126
851858LV00006B/124